# DLPA

## TO END CHRONIC PAIN AND DEPRESSION

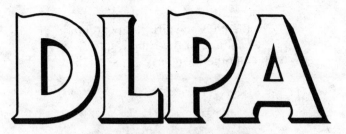

# DLPA

# TO END CHRONIC PAIN AND DEPRESSION

BY ARNOLD FOX, M.D.
AND BARRY FOX
FOREWORD BY LENDON SMITH, M.D.

LONG SHADOW BOOKS
PUBLISHED BY POCKET BOOKS NEW YORK

To the boys and girls in my group,
Scouting For the Handicapped,
and all others who say "yes" to life.

Another *Original* publication of LONG SHADOW BOOKS

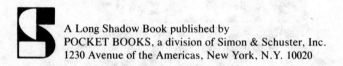

A Long Shadow Book published by
POCKET BOOKS, a division of Simon & Schuster, Inc.
1230 Avenue of the Americas, New York, N.Y. 10020

ISBN: 0-671-54503-5

First Long Shadow Books printing February, 1985

10 9 8 7 6 5 4

LONG SHADOW BOOKS and colophon are
trademarks of Simon & Schuster, Inc.

Printed in the U.S.A.

# WARNING

Although the clinical research (my own and others) and the laboratory studies on DL-phenylalanine (DLPA) indicate that it is safe and effective *when used as I have outlined in this book,* as a physician I recommend that anyone considering starting on the DLPA Program (or any other program) consult his or her physician.

I recommend against using DLPA during pregnancy or lactation. Pregnant or lactating women should not expose the fetus or newborn to *anything* except their normal diet. It is best to be safe. Neither should any person suffering from the genetic disease phenylketonuria (PKU) take DLPA—they cannot metabolize phenylalanine normally. This also applies to those on a phenylalanine-restricted diet.

Neither do I recommend the use of DLPA for children under the age of 14. I arbitrarily chose this age because as an internist and cardiologist I do not usually treat children. However, physicians experienced in treating children may wish to examine the DLPA literature.

Although the information presented in the case histories is true, names and identifying information have been changed.

# ACKNOWLEDGMENTS

There are many people to thank for helping Barry and me prepare this book. First and foremost is my wife, Hannah, who shepherded this book through the writing process: reading, editing, correcting, and helping to polish the manuscript. Her cheerful encouragement and hard work kept us going. And thanks to my children: Howard, our new lawyer, for typing and correcting the manuscript; Robin, for reading and commenting on the book; Steven, our soon-to-be lawyer, for challenging us at every point; Eric, our new M.D., for late-night discussions and reviews; Barbara, my beautiful and helpful daughter; and Bruce Hiam, our youngest, whose interest and encouragement in our effort never flagged. Last, but certainly not least, is Barry, my coauthor and soon-to-be Ph.D. It seems like only yesterday he was a little boy, but here he is today, discussing subtle issues of biochemistry and physiology with me. And thanks to the rest of my "family": Carlos and Anna Marie Cueva, Michael Cohen, and especially Mercedes Cohen for her timely assistance.

I owe a debt of gratitude to my office staff, Shirley Feldman and Jeanne Schwartz, who have taken such excellent care of my patients over the years. I am also in debt to those who gave their time to read the manuscript: my old Army buddy, Herb Gooberman, and his wife Bernice; Eleanor Steinberg; Shari Schneider; Alice Kaye. (And Shelly Stoll—because I promised.)

I have been fortunate to be able to draw on the talent, experience, writings, and inspiration of many fellow professionals: Linus Pauling, M.D., Richard Wurtman, M.D., Lendon Smith, M.D., Earl Mindell, Ph.D., A. A. Chaplin, M.D., Mel Bircoll, M.D., the Reverend Dan Morgan, the Reverend Dale Batesole, Joseph Bark, M.D., Richard Huemer, M.D., William Goldwag, M.D., Uzie Reiss, M.D., John Libeskind, M.D., U.C.L.A.'s marvelous teacher and researcher, and many others, including researchers in the fields of brain biochemistry and endorphins. And, of course, Harry Kaye, for freeing me to pursue my studies.

My special thanks to AminoLabs for generously supplying me with DLPA used in my studies; to Rex Maughan and Cliff Evarts of Forever Living Products, Inc., of Arizona, for providing me with aloe vera for use in the clinical studies, and to Ethical Nutrients of Laguna Beach, California.

Finally, my warmest thanks to all my patients, who have taught me so much about life, health, and faith.

# CONTENTS

# FOREWORD
## by Lendon Smith, M.D.

Dr. Arnold Fox and I have shared many podia, and I have found that we also share a desire to help people without hurting them. By that I mean we want to relieve our patients' problems without resorting to drugs and procedures that can harm them. My experience in pediatrics and his in internal medicine have led us to attempt to find the reasons for people's illness, rather than simply treating the symptoms willy-nilly as they arise. I learned to stop drugging hyperactive children because nutritional and other methods are superior, and better for the child. Dr. Fox learned to open clogged blood vessels in his patients by means of diet and other methods, and fewer drugs and surgeries.

But he has found, as I have, that a program of nutrition and exercise is not the full and complete answer to every sickness and pain in the world. Some people are stuck with destructive genes that pull them down; some have had accidents that left scar tissue pinching nerves; some have problems we doctors cannot diagnose; some cannot absorb enough of the nutrients they eat to keep themselves free of disease. I believe many people suffering from pain or disease will do anything to feel better. They take drugs, often becoming hooked. They drink to forget their miseries and depression.

New research has indicated that a great deal of chronic pain and depression is due to the victim's inability to produce enough of certain brain chemicals. This exciting research has hinted at new methods of dealing with pain and depression without using drugs that can harm our patients. If you cannot get rid of your pain and are tired of aspirin; if everyone wants you to see a psychiatrist because they are convinced your problem is "all in your head'', this book should really help you break out of the pain–depression–pain cycle once and for all.

Dr. Fox has combined nutrition, exercise, a positive mental outlook, and DL-phenylalanine (DLPA) into a natural approach to relieving pain and depression. He attacks the problems from many directions simultaneously. This is a sound, realistic, and natural approach to the very serious problems of chronic pain and depression.

I have tried DLPA myself. And come to think of it, the ache in my back is better.

# 1

# DLPA: MODERN HEALTH PHENOMENON

The most important and exciting scientific discovery of our time was made 12 years ago at the Johns Hopkins University School of Medicine. Thanks to that breakthrough and the research that followed, we are on the threshold of a new age in medicine. Much of the debilitating chronic pain and depression that now afflict us may soon be nothing but an unpleasant memory.

In 1972 Dr. Candace Pert and Dr. Solomon Snyder showed that morphine (a powerful painkilling drug) fits into certain nerve cell structures in the brain like a key fits its lock.[1] In other words, morphine can unlock previously unknown powers of the brain. But this was a puzzling discovery: Why do human brain cells have specific structures that interact with morphine? These two scientists, along with others, proposed a simple but radical explanation: The human brain must produce its own form of morphine!

## ENDORPHINS = *ENDOGENOUS MORPHINE*

Studies at major universities around the world have shown that the brain does in fact produce many hormone-like chemicals that bear a close functional resemblance to morphine. These morphinelike chemicals are called endorphins (*end*ogenous mor*phine*) because they are produced by the body (are endogenous), and are similar to morphine.

11

## MORPHINE FOR THE BRAIN?

Why does the brain make endorphins and what are they used for? With a bold leap of scientific imagination, researchers hypothesized that the endorphins might be part of a natural, built-in pain-control system.

The human body is an intricate and beautifully designed series of checks and balances. Why shouldn't we have a pain-control network to regulate pain perception?

## THE MOST POWERFUL PAINKILLERS KNOWN . . .

Pain researchers began testing the endorphins by administering them to experimental animals and to human pain patients. The results surprised and impressed patients and researchers alike: The endorphins were much more powerful than morphine, the strongest painkiller we have. One of the endorphins, beta-endorphin, was 18 to 50 times more effective than morphine. Another endorphin, called dynorphin, was *over 500 times stronger than morphine* in some biological tests.

## . . . CAN'T BE USED . . .

Are the endorphins the ultimate painkillers? Unfortunately, the answer is yes—and no. For reasons I'll discuss in later chapters, using the endorphins themselves as drugs to control chronic pain is impractical, inefficient, costly, and sometimes even dangerous. But scientists refused to give up on the endorphins. There had to be a way to get them to work for us.

## THE ENDORPHINS NEED AN ASSIST

Dr. Seymour Ehrenpreis thought he had an answer. Dr. Ehrenpreis, a pharmacologist at the Chicago Medical School, injected laboratory animals with a nutrient he hoped would raise endorphin levels and block pain. It worked—but that was only the beginning. Besides raising endorphin levels and blocking pain, the nutrient was nontoxic and nonaddictive. That made it superior to all other known painkillers. Moreover, this nutrient worked *with* other painkillers, and actually became stronger with repeated use. It gave the endorphins the assist they needed to relieve pain. The results of Dr. Ehrenpreis's and other studies suggested we were dealing with a substance that would revolutionize pain therapy.

## EXOTIC WONDER DRUG?

The substance is not a drug at all, but a simple nutritional amino acid called phenylalanine (PA). The successful studies involved D-phenylalanine (DPA) or DL-phenylalanine (DLPA), both of which are forms of PA. This book is concerned with the DLPA form of PA.

DL-phenylalanine is not a drug: It does not actually block pain itself. DL-phenylalanine works by protecting your own naturally produced endorphins, effectively extending their life span in the nervous system. DL-phenylalanine helps your body heal itself.

## DLPA RELIEVES PAIN—AND MORE

DL-phenylalanine is also a powerful, safe antidepressant. In several clinical studies DLPA has proven to be as effective as commonly prescribed antidepressant drugs. And it does not have the side effects of these drugs. The 10 million people seriously disabled by depression can join the 70 million people who are crippled by chronic pain and arthritis in looking to DLPA for relief.

In addition, DLPA helps relieve the symptoms of premenstrual syndrome (PMS), reduces the swelling and inflammation of arthritis, and enhances the effects of acupuncture. Working through the brain, DLPA can relieve some of the symptoms of other diseases as well.

DL-phenylalanine is now being used clinically around the United States and by many thousands of people who suffer from chronic pain and/or depression. The dramatic results indicate that we finally have a safe, wonderfully effective weapon with which we can conquer chronic pain and depression.

In this book, the general public and practicing health professionals will for the first time be given an understandable review of the DLPA phenomenon. I am not trying to present an exhaustive study of esoteric scientific literature, but a balance of up-to-date scientific knowledge those who have no scientific background can understand.

More scientific study is needed, but all indications are that with DLPA, chronic pain and depression can be effectively controlled by a safe nutritional substance.

# 2

# CHRONIC PAIN

*Pain is a more terrible lord of mankind than even death himself.*

—ALBERT SCHWEITZER

"I can't stand it anymore! Since the car accident five years ago, the pain is like a vise. All day long, at night, everytime I move I get this excruciating pain in my back! I've been to every doctor in town. I've had surgeries and pills up to my neck. They don't help. This pain won't go away!"

Pain is the giant fist crushing your lower back, the jackhammer pounding into your skull, the invisible force twisting your fingers and hands into grotesque and useless configurations, the fire burning in your joints and muscles. Pain is the phenomenon sending an estimated seventy million Americans to their doctors every year. Pain is an albatross around our individual and collective necks, crippling our lives and aspirations, and, in many cases, subverting our desire to live.

Human beings have unwillingly shared a very intimate relationship with pain since well before our ancestors began to walk on two legs. Ours is indeed a pained nation. We spend billions of dollars on analgesics (painkillers) and therapies of every description—to no avail. We have tried every imaginable remedy in our battle against pain, but it seems as if the "magic pain pill" is but a wisp of the imagination. How serious is the pain problem in this country?

- 70 million Americans are racked by back pain;
- 36 million are afflicted with arthritis;
- 20 million are tortured by migraine headaches, and
- 800,000 have cancer pain, the most excruciating pain of all.[1]

Knowing that one out of every three people in this country is a pain statistic is not much comfort if you are one of those three.

- Every year we spend $4 billion on migraine medications.
- Sixty-five million workdays are lost every year to those migraine headaches.
- One in seven of us has arthritis.
- Every year we lose well over 150 million workdays to chronic pain.
- The direct medical costs for lower back pain total $5 billion a year.
- The total bill for chronic pain and arthritis—direct and indirect costs—comes to well over $50 billion every year!

And the human suffering involved is too immense to measure.

## WE'RE NOT CURING PAIN

But this is the twentieth century. We can send men to the moon. Surely we have some good pain pills. Yes, we have all kinds of pills for pain. There's aspirin, Tylenol, Parafon Forte, Percocet-5, Phenaphen with codeine, Ascriptin, Bufferin, Cama Inlay, A.P.C. with codeine, Equagesic, Fiorinal, Midol, Ascriptin with codeine, Demerol, Empracet with codeine, Hydromorphone, Meperidine, Numorphan, Percodan, Percogesic, Darvocet, oxycodone, Talwin, Tegretol . . . that is just the short list. These are powerful and potentially dangerous drugs, especially the narcotics. And if the pills do not help you, you can try any of many types of surgery, or biofeedback, hypnosis, acupuncture, counseling, and other techniques.

But to be perfectly honest, we doctors cannot cure most of the pain our patients suffer from. Our pills are not always safe or effective. The typical pain patient goes from doctor to doctor looking for relief we cannot give them.

Ellen O., a 45-year-old mother of three, first came to see me five years ago. Her complaint was chronic, unendurable lower back pain.

"You know how you crack a nut open by squeezing it in a nutcracker?" she asked. "That's how my back feels all the time. Like someone's trying to crack it open. This goes on all day. I can't think, I can't do anything!"

Ellen tried every pill in her medicine chest, all the pills in her friends' medicine chests, then went to a doctor. Failing to find anything physically wrong with her, he prescribed stronger pain pills, tranquilizers for her nerves, and told her to call him if she did not feel better in a few weeks. A month later she called to say she felt worse than ever so he sent her to a specialist. The specialist examined her, but found nothing physically wrong with her back. He gave her very powerful narcotic painkillers and more tranquilizers.

By now Ellen was a walking pharmacy. In her purse she carried five different (mostly narcotic) anti-pain pills and two tranquilizers. She took pep pills to keep herself awake because the other pills made her so sleepy. She was hooked. She could not get through the day without taking at least a dozen pills. And her back? It hurt as much as ever.

Cursing the doctors who could not cure her pain, muttering darkly about the unfairness of life, Ellen sank into a deep depression. Her family and friends were sympathetic when the trouble started. But by now they suspected Ellen was faking the pain to get attention. Even her doctors tactfully suggested she see a psychiatrist.

Ellen is the typical pain patient stumbling blindly down the pain path. With each step she sank further into the bogs of drugs, depression, and addiction. And always more pain. Conventional medicine had little to offer Ellen, save this choice: learn to live with the pain, or be so drugged up you can barely function. Ellen opted for the second, becoming a drugged, depressed zombie, blindly groping her way through a hazy fog she knew as life.

It's not much of a choice. It is very frustrating for me, as a physician, to have to stand by helplessly, watching chronic pain destroy lives. It's maddening to know that for many patients, an hour, or even a few minutes without pain is like a gift from heaven.

## DES AND OTHER PATENTED POISONS

Yes, we have a lot of pain pills, and some of them are pretty strong. Especially the narcotics. *But they are all dangerous— every one of them—even the ubiquitous aspirin tablet.* So many of the pills we blithely swallow wreak havoc on our bodies. Every so often a drug is banned, but the majority of patented poisons remain on the pharmacists' shelves.

Diethylstilbesterol (DES) was a popular poison given to pregnant women. Diethylstilbesterol was an effective treatment for the women, but it gave a lot of their soon-to-be-born daughters cancer (and some sons as well). This was a psychologically cruel cancer, appearing often or not appearing until the daughters were in their teens and twenties, and beginning to consider having their own children.

Then there is the brief story of Oroflex, an arthritis medication. It used to be that when a drug company developed a new drug it would inform the medical profession. Doctors would then evaluate the drug and decide if they wanted to prescribe it for their patients. That changed very recently when the drug companies decided to go right to the people. They began holding press conferences to announce their great new wonder drugs.

In the spring of 1983 a major drug company held a press conference to tell the American people about Oroflex. Arthritis patients immediately rushed to their doctors asking for a prescription. One of my patients, a 35-year-old woman with rheumatoid arthritis, came to my office demanding a prescription for Oroflex. I refused, saying that it had not been on the market long enough for me to see what side effects it had. I told her to ignore what the drug company's advertising department said and wait to see what side effects develop. That was in May of 1983. In July of the same year she called and told me she had gone to another doctor and received a prescription for Oroflex. It helped her arthritis, but there was a problem: her fingernails were growing away from her fingers at a 90-degree angle. That is, if she held her fingers vertically, her fingernails were horizontal. She's lucky that was her only problem. By then we knew that Oroflex, which had been legal in Britain for some time, killed many people who took it. It seems that when the drug company was applying for permission to sell Oroflex in this country, they forgot to tell our Food and Drug Administration (FDA) about those deaths over in Britain. (The FDA does *not* test drugs. It allows the drug companies to conduct their own tests, then studies the results *provided by the drug companies*. I am not accusing anybody of cheating—they just forgot.) By August, 1983, Oroflex had disappeared from pharmacists' shelves in this country.

How about some of the drugs that remain on the market? How safe are they?

- INDOCIN—I have been called upon countless times to examine the inside of a patient's stomach or esophagus with a gastroscope. Many of these patients have had their intestinal lining badly damaged by this arthritis drug. If it is prolonged enough, this kind of damage can, and will, kill you.

- PERCODAN—I have seen side effects such as dizziness, nausea, vomiting, and constipation, among others. This painkiller's worst side effect is addiction. (Percodan's major ingredient is a semisynthetic narcotic.) When I first came to Los Angeles in the 1950s, doctors were handing out Percodan like candy, and I was constantly seeing patients who were addicted to it. The government finally stepped in and required the use of special triplicate prescription forms for this drug. The patient takes two copies to the pharmacist, who will not give out Percodan unless he or she gets both forms. One copy is then sent by the pharmacist to the appropriate government agency so they can keep track of how much Percodan each doctor gives out. Mandatory use of this form has cut Percodan addiction considerably.

- TALWIN—The side effects I have seen from this painkiller include nausea, vomiting, diarrhea, fainting, headaches, dizziness, sweating, and rash. The medical literature contains warnings about possible adverse reactions such as lowered blood pressure, depression, and other serious problems. In years past I saw many people addicted to Talwin.

And what of aspirin, that ever-popular panacea? Is it as harmless as we have been led to believe?

• ASPIRIN—If you put a gastroscope into a person's stomach you can watch as aspirin irritates every part of the stomach lining it touches. Heavy aspirin users generally bleed internally over long periods of time. Because the bleeding is slow and steady the stool will not be noticeably discolored, but a laboratory analysis of the stool will show that it does contain appreciable amounts of blood.

I have seen all kinds of side effects attributable to pain pills: nausea, diarrhea, vomiting, constipation, bloating, dizziness, headaches, depression, hallucinations, poor vision, elevated blood pressure, lowered blood pressure, poor circulation, anxiety, mood changes, respiratory depression, blood clots, ulcers, bleeding stomachs, and irregular heart rhythms.

Which is worse: the pain or the cure?

I am not suggesting that every drug on the market should be banned. Many drugs work well, and not everyone will suffer horrendous side effects. For some people the side effects are less dangerous or painful than the original problem. And most drugs are not like DES or Oroflex, because most drugs have been fairly and honestly tested. But the fact remains that every single drug, including aspirin, has potentially serious side effects. And I mean *every* drug.

## CONDEMNED TO SUFFER?

Must we endure the relentless stabbing, crushing, twisting, deadening, and maddening effects of chronic pain? Are our choices restricted to learning to live with the pain, being so doped up we can't think, or risking serious side effects?

I don't believe so. The initiation rites for young males of the Mandian Indian tribe in the Dakota region included an excruciating torture. Young initiates were hung from the rafters by knives stuck through their hands. The braves-to-be hung for several hours before being cut down, and silently watched as two fingers of their left hand were swiftly cut off. No anesthetics or other pain remedies were allowed, but the young men withstood this ordeal. And historical records boast of badly wounded soldiers who continued to fight, unaware of and unhampered by their serious wounds. Like the Indian braves, the soldiers passed off pain that would destroy you or me. How? With their endorphins, their built-in pain-control system.

## WHAT'S THE CATCH?

OK, the endorphins are terrific painkillers, they are made by the body, and they helped the Indians and soldiers withstand horrible pain. What's the catch? If the endorphins are so great, how come seventy million Americans are tortured by chronic pain? Do you have to be half-dead before your endorphins do anything for you?

The answer to this somewhat complex question will be dealt with in several sections of the book, but our chronic pain problem may be due to a breakdown in the endorphin system. What causes this breakdown? Stress!

## STRESS IS THE CATCH

Repeated physical pain and emotional upset can cause stress. Dr. Hans Selye has shown that the body responds to stress by mobilizing its resources to protect itself. That's why the Indian braves and soldiers could withstand their pain. But if the battle against stress is too difficult, or prolonged beyond a certain variable point, the body will weaken, run out of resources and eventually fail. The brain releases endorphins as part of the reaction to stress—but the supply is limited. Although prolific and resilient, the human body can only do so much. Chronic stress may simply overwhelm your ability to manufacture sufficient endorphins. With fewer and fewer endorphins available, you are more and more likely to fall prey to pain. I believe that many of the chronic pain patients in this country are suffering from a stress-induced lack of endorphins. In chapter 11 I'll discuss some of the studies linking chronic pain (a stressful condition) to low endorphin levels.

## ASSISTING THE ENDORPHINS WITH DLPA

Your body makes endorphins. It also makes enzymes that "chew up" the endorphins, making them useless for killing pain. Meanwhile, stress is depleting your endorphin stores. Researchers tried helping pain patients by giving them injections of "extra" endorphins, but the procedures are impractical, costly, and in some cases too dangerous for all but the most hopeless pain cases.

Was that the end of the endorphin story? No. In 1978 a nutrient called DLPA breathed new life into the endorphins and ushered in an exciting new era in the history of pain relief. Study after study has shown that DLPA effectively "protects" the endorphins from the endorphin-chewing enzymes, giving them more time to block pain. In test after test DLPA has proven to be a very effective and safe pain killer. DLPA may very well be the answer to chronic pain.

## DLPA = DL-PHENYLALANINE

DLPA is a nutrient, not a drug. It is a form of a common amino acid, called phenylalanine, found in the foods we eat. Phenylalanine (PA) is an essential amino acid which comes in two forms: D-phenylalanine (DPA) and L-phenylalanine (LPA). The two forms are mirror images of each other, like your right and left hands. DPA is the "right handed" form, while LPA is the "left-handed" form.

DL-phenylalanine is a 50/50 mixture of DPA and LPA. L-phenylalanine has nutritional value, and D-phenylalanine has painkilling and depression-lifting properties. DL-phenylalanine, the 50/50 mixture, has both nutritional *and* therapeutic value.

DL-phenylalanine is not an endorphin; it does not, in itself, block pain. It works by slowing down the activity of the "endorphin-chewing" enzymes in your body. DL-phenylalanine extends the lifespan of your painkilling endorphins.

The following abbreviations are used:

Phenylalanine = PA, or "the amino acid"
D-phenylalanine = DPA, or D-PA, or "the D-form"
L-phenylalanine = LPA, or L-PA, or "the L-form"

Phenylalanine is pronounced "feen-el-ala-neen."

## SAFE AND EFFECTIVE

In all my 28 years of studying and practicing medicine I have never been so impressed by a therapeutic phenomenon as DLPA represents. I have seen pain firsthand. I have treated patients whose pain was so intense it destroyed them. Modern medicine has held out no hope for many chronic pain patients. For the millions and millions of Americans conventional pain therapy has failed to help, DLPA gives hope. Is DLPA the "magic pain pill" we have been looking for? Present evidence indicates it might be. It is certainly much better than anything else we have. Let's compare DLPA to aspirin and narcotics:

|  | Aspirin | Narcotics | DLPA |
|---|---|---|---|
| Duration of Action | 2-6 hrs | 2-8 hrs | 24-270 hrs |
| Does Tolerance Develop? | Yes | Yes | No |
| Can Addiction Result? | Yes | Yes | No |
| Adverse Side Effects? | Yes | Yes | No |
| Toxic To Humans? | Yes | Yes | No |

Because DLPA works by protecting your natural endorphins, it is very safe and effective. It's also long-lasting, non-addictive, has no adverse side effects, and is non-toxic.

## IS DLPA SAFE?

DLPA is extraordinarily safe and remarkably free of adverse side effects. The FDA (Food and Drug Administration) considers DLPA to be a Nutrient/Dietary Supplement. (See Code of Federal Regulations, Title 21, Section 582.5590) DL-phenylalanine is on the federal government's Generally Recognized As Safe (GRAS) list—the various drugs are not. Here is a graph comparing the toxicity of DLPA to some common pain pills. As you can see, DL-phenylalanine barely makes it onto the graph:

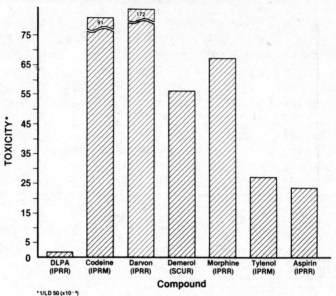

ACUTE TOXICITY OF DL-PHENYLALANINE
COMPARED WITH COMMONLY USED
ANALGESIC DRUGS

*1/LD 50 (x10⁻⁴)

## DLPA LASTS A LONG TIME

Conventional pain pills do not work for very long. They have to be taken over and over again, usually several times a day. For example:

• Darvon is usually taken every 4 hours.
• Demerol is usually taken every 3 to 4 hours.
• Percodan is usually taken every 6 hours.
• Aspirin lasts up to 6 hours.

• *DLPA works for approximately five days!*
(even longer when taken *with* aspirin)

Here is a graphic demonstration of the difference:

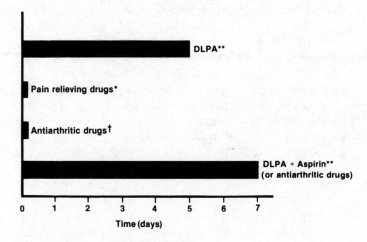

**AVERAGE DURATION OF ACTION OF DLPA
COMPARED TO PAIN RELIEVING DRUGS AND
ANTIARTHRITIC DRUGS**

*Average of 5 commonly prescribed analgesic drugs
†Average of 5 commonly prescribed antiarthritic drugs
**Estimate based on published values and clinical experience.

We don't know exactly why DLPA works so well with aspirin. They appear to attack pain in two ways simultaneously:

1. The endorphins seem to regulate pain; DLPA protects the endorphins, thereby reducing pain.
2. Aspirin decreases the production of prostaglandins, which are hormones that seem to promote pain.

So, taking DLPA with aspirin pushes the pain "break pedal," and takes pressure off the pain "accelerator." This is the theory proposed by Dr. Ehrenpreis, who conducted the original phenylalanine/pain studies, to explain why DLPA and aspirin work so well together.

## DLPA—AN ALTERNATIVE

In later chapters I'll discuss DLPA, the endorphins, and pain in greater detail. If you are interested, skip ahead to chapters 11 and 12 for more details. But for now, let's see how DLPA and my DLPA Anti-Pain Plan has helped people.

Edith D., a 35-year-old lawyer, had been on massive doses of aspirin and other drugs for treatment of lower back pain. I first saw her when her doctor asked me to do a gastroscopy to check her stomach for ulcerations.

I passed the gastroscope through her mouth into her stomach. It was raw and bleeding from the aspirin and other drugs. I reported my findings to her doctor. He said he would give her a new medicine, this one to help her bloody stomach.

"More medicine?" I said. "How about if we give her less medicine?"

"What?"

"The aspirin is ruining her stomach, and it's not helping her pain much. The new medicine may or may not help her stomach, but we know it's going to have some other side effect that will require yet another medicine, and another, and another. Let's break the cycle. Instead of more, let's give her less medicine."

"Dr. Fox," he said, "I've heard all about how you feel about vitamins and nutrition, but this is real medicine. I'm a physician. I deal with facts."

"Take a look in Edith's stomach and you'll see some facts." We finally agreed to go with less medicine.

When I told Edith, she said, "Good. I've had enough of those damned drugs that don't do anything but make me sicker. When this started I just had pain.Now I'm vomiting blood!"

Her doctor and I agreed that dealing with all of her problems except the pain would be easy because they were all side effects to the medicines. I put her on a version of my DLPA Anti-Pain Plan, carefully reducing, then eliminating her medications. All the problems except the pain quickly vanished. I got her to give up her junk-food diet and start eating the kinds of foods I describe in the next chapter, and put her on

DLPA. Within two weeks her pain was significantly reduced. Two more weeks and it was almost completely gone. The next step was to convince Edith to cut back on her stressful lifestyle and give her endorphins system a chance to recuperate.

Now Edith is on an on/off schedule with DLPA, one week on and three weeks off. (DL-phenylalanine continues working after you have stopped taking it, so you do not have to take it every day.) Edith says her pain has been reduced dramatically.

## FIFTEEN YEARS OF CHRONIC PAIN

Mrs. R. N. came from Florida to see me after reading an article I wrote on pain. At the age of 30 she was in an auto accident that left her in great pain "all of the time." Now 45 years old, she had spent the last 15 years going to internists, neurologists, neurosurgeons, orthopedists, and anesthesiologists. She had had nerve blocks (injections into her back), surgery on her back twice, ultrasound, and other healing modalities. She saw chiropractors, acupuncturists, naturopaths, and psychologists. All of these professionals had done their best, and they had all helped her, but only for a little while.

She was brought to my office in a wheelchair because walking was too difficult. Opening a lunch bag filled with a colorful array of pills, tablets, and potions, she dumped the contents onto my desk and said, "I've got every size, shape, and color." She smiled. "I'd be eternally grateful if you could give me some relief from this pain."

She needed handfuls of pills every day to dull the pain and anxiety, plus sleeping pills at night. The medicines made her feel "numb all the time, like a big blob." She was also sad because she felt she was such a burden on her husband and children.

After taking a complete history and doing a physical examination, plus the first day's round of tests, I started her on my DLPA Anti-Pain Plan. I made several adjustments in the plan specific to her very severe pain. She was staying at a nearby hotel and agreed to come to my office every day so I could monitor her progress.

The initial response was slow in coming. Ten days passed before she reported a small reduction in her pain. I increased her DLPA dosage. By the end of the second week she was jubilant!

"It's really going away!" she exclaimed. By the end of the third week she was out of her wheelchair and was sleeping the entire night through without taking sleeping pills. By the end of the fourth week she was able to exercise (walk) and had begun to lose weight, which helped her self-esteem. She described her pain as "75 percent gone. I'm a person again," she said.

She returned to Florida. I called her local doctor and he agreed to slowly reduce her medication and keep her on my DLPA Anti-Pain Plan. I still hear from her a couple of times a year. She's doing very well. There's still a little pain, but "nothing I can't manage. DL-phenylalanine is all I need. I don't have to take those drugs anymore." When I last heard she was a part-time volunteer in a pain-relief center in Florida, giving others hope by sharing her story.

## FROM LION-LIKE TO LIFE-LIKE

One of my most delightful experiences with DLPA did not involve chronic pain. Instead, the patient was suffering from Parkinson's Disease, a disorder of movement centers in the brain. Voluntary control of movement is upset; groups of muscles twitch uncontrollably, other muscles become stiff and sluggish, or even paralyzed.

Alfonso M. is a 70-year-old businessman who first showed signs of Parkinson's at age 60. Otherwise in good health, he developed the characteristic twitching of the hands. His symptoms progressed slowly, and for several years his medication seemed to control the disease. In any case, he was able to continue working and his spirits were high.

Then his condition deteriorated. Within six months he was barely able to walk. Muscles all over his body became rigid (cog wheel rigidity). His face was "lionlike"; he drooled and had no expression in his face because he could not move any of his facial muscles. (Facial paralysis is characteristic of this disease.) Before many more months passed he was almost completely paralyzed. He lay in a hospital bed all day, unable to feed himself, drooling, having to urinate into a tube, not even able to change the channel of the television set he watched.

Alfonso became depressed, apathetic, and withdrawn, waiting to die. As far as he was concerned, the sooner he died the better.

Without disturbing his other medication, I put him on DLPA. Within three weeks his rigid muscles began to loosen. Soon he was able to walk; it was difficult, but he could walk. His facial and other muscles relaxed enough for him to stop drooling, feed himself, write, and move around a bit. The most encouraging change, however, was in his attitude. He recaptured his enthusiasm, his interest in life and in the future. He talked about business plans, his upcoming trip, and his family, all with renewed interest. He wanted to keep living!

Now that we have learned a little about DLPA and pain, let's see how Dr. Fox's DLPA Anti-Pain Plan can help you.

# 3

# DR. FOX'S DLPA ANTIPAIN PLAN

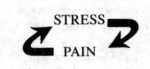

Pain fuels stress, stress energizes pain.

Robert F. was a 25-year-old high-school teacher who had not known a pain-free day for 3 years. For 3 years, ever since he started teaching, every movement of his jaw had been accented by a "sledgehammer hitting right below my ear." The several specialists who found nothing physically wrong with his jaw gave Robert pain pills and tranquilizers.

Robert is a highly stressed individual. Vaguely aware of the relationship between stress and his pain, he ignored it. "I like the feeling of blood racing through my veins," he said. "It makes me feel strong." He loved stress—his jaw hated it. The more he stressed himself the more his jaw hurt. Although he did not recognize it, his job contributed a great deal to his stress load (the pain began when he left college and began teaching). One of his co-workers, also a patient of mine, said to me: "I hope he stresses himself so much his jaw falls off. Then we won't have to listen to him and his stress anymore."

## EXERCISE IN FUTILITY

The point of Robert's story is this: If stress is causing your pain, it is generally futile to take pain pills. The medicine will help some, but stress is stronger than pain pills. And the pills have side effects. Skip the pills and get to the root of the problem—stress. It is all right to use the pills as a temporary measure until you beat the stress. But don't fall into the pill pit, taking more and stronger pills all the time. A warehouse full of pills would not have helped Robert. No conventional pain therapy would be likely to relieve this man's pain—short of severing all the nerves in half his face. That would take care of the pain in his jaw, but the stress would turn on another part of his body with equal fury.

Robert's case is typical; not in the particulars, but in the sense that stress is the villain. Dealing with this kind of problem requires a two-edged sword; one edge to dispatch pain and one to destroy stress. Dr. Fox's DLPA Antipain Plan relieves pain and reduces stress simultaneously.

## ONE PILL . . . THREE TIMES A DAY

This is the basic DLPA antipain schedule I start my pain patients on:

*375 Milligrams of DLPA Three Times a Day*

375 milligrams with breakfast
375 milligrams with lunch
375 milligrams with dinner

I instruct my patients to have regular meals: breakfast at 8:00 A.M., lunch at noon, and dinner between 5 and 6 P.M. DL-phenylalanine (DLPA) should be taken with the meal, or within an hour after completing the meal. I prefer it to be taken five minutes after finishing the meal.

On the third day, if no pain relief has occurred, I generally have them increase the dosage to:

*750 Milligrams of DLPA Three Times a Day*

750 mg with breakfast
750 mg with lunch
750 mg with dinner

If my patients have trouble sleeping at night because DLPA gives them a feeling of excitement or energy, I have them cut the dinner dose in half.

NOTE: *You do not have to stop taking any medication prescribed by your doctor to benefit from DLPA. In fact, DLPA can greatly enhance the effectiveness of aspirin and analgesic drugs.*

This is the basic plan, which I vary to meet the needs of individual patients. I carefully monitor their progress adjusting the dosage up or down as needed.

*I tell my patients to stay with DLPA—give it a chance to work.* My observation has been that it generally takes anywhere from two days to three weeks for DLPA to take effect. In a few cases, it may take as long as four to six weeks before it works, so I tell my patients not to get discouraged. DL-phenylalanine is not fast-acting, like aspirin; it takes *at least* one day to have an effect. Give it a chance to work!

 When they have felt really good for a full week, I have my patients stop taking DLPA and wait for the symptoms to recur. They go on an alternating schedule, taking DLPA until they feel good for a full week, then not taking it until the symptoms recur, and so on. Many of my patients only use DLPA one out of every three or four weeks. Patients are encouraged to adjust their dosage in consultation with their physician.

DL-phenylalanine and aspirin: I have some of my patients taking DLPA and aspirin together. If they were already taking aspirin, I have them continue taking it while taking DLPA. The two work well together, enhancing each other's effectiveness.

CAUTION: *I recommend against using DLPA during pregnancy or lactation. Pregnant or lactating women should not expose the fetus or newborn to anything except their normal diet. It is best to be safe. Neither should any person suffering from the genetic disease phenyketonuria (PKU) take DLPA—they cannot metabolize phenylalanine normally. This also applies to those on a phenylalanine restricted diet. Consult your doctor. Neither do I recommend the use of DLPA for children under the age of 14. I arbitrarily chose this age because as an internist and cardiologist I do not usually treat children. However, physicians experienced in treating children may wish to examine the DLPA literature. They may find an appropriate use for DLPA in children, such as in cases of juvenile rheumatoid arthritis.*

## NOT MEGADOSES

I'd like to stress that the dosage levels I recommend to my patients *are not megadoses.* Even at the higher level (750 milligrams three times a day) it only comes to 2,250 milligrams a day. This yields just about 100 percent of the daily phenylalanine requirement suggested by the research of Dr. William Rose at the University of Illinois (see chapter 12). This is relatively little when compared to the large doses (many times the recommended daily allowance) of vitamins and minerals routinely taken. Not only that, but when you are on an on/off schedule your average daily intake is much lower, dropping by 50 to 75 percent.

## THE FOUNDATION OF MENTAL BLUEPRINTS

In medical school we physicians are taught to separate the mind and body. We are told to deal with the body and treat its diseases. I believe this is the wrong approach. The mind is part of the body, the body is part of the mind. One cannot be torn from the other.

The body has arms and legs, eyes and ears with which to contact and manipulate the world. It has internal organs that pump blood, process chemicals, build and transport materials. Then there is the brain, the control room, command center, clearing house, library, and research laboratory. The brain is in constant communication with all other parts of the body. It continually converts intangible, phantomlike thoughts into tangible, real chemicals that regularly alter the course of your health and life. (I will talk more about this in chapter 14.)

Your mind mirrors your world. Acting through your eyes, ears, nose, fingers, and other sensors, the brain takes in information and turns it into thoughts and emotions. The physical counterpart of your feelings and emotions are the chemical messengers sent through your body.

When your mind is angry your foot is angry. When your mind laughs your lungs laugh. When your mind cries your stomach cries. When your mind smiles your heart smiles. When your mind feels anything, you—the entire you, mind and body—also feel it. That is what I mean when I say the body is the mind and the mind is the body. They are so intertwined any attempt to separate them is ludicrous and even dangerous.

The foundation for your castle of pain-free living begins with Mental Blueprints. Mental Blueprints are the instructions etched into your mind. They determine what kind of messages your brain sends to the rest of your body—messages of health or messages of disease. Stress causes the brain to send out diseased messages, so you want to keep stress out of your mind.

Stress-free living begins with this simple message written onto your Mental Blueprints. It is a short sentence that speaks volumes:

**Belief Is the Power of the Mind.**

The kind of messages your brain sends to the rest of your body is determined by your brain's interpretation of your world. If your mind accepts something as stressful, the entire body reacts to that stress. What the mind believes, the body feels.

Think and you shall feel! Good thoughts or bad thoughts, they will be reflected in the health or disease of your body. As the great researcher René Dubos said: "Whatever happens in the mind of man is always reflected in the disease of his body."

## SAY AND SEE YOUR PAIN AWAY

The key, then, is to believe you are not stressed. The brain is a marvelously receptive instrument. It believes what you tell it. If you tell your brain you are stressed, your brain tells the rest of your body to get stressed. But if you tell your brain you are not stressed the brain passes the good word on.

That is where affirmations come in. Affirmations are used to tell your brain and the rest of your body that you are not stressed.

I believe that affirmations are the most important tool you have for changing your thoughts and your life. The way you react to your world is determined by the words, thoughts, and ideas zipping around your mind.

- Affirmations are a way of putting only the most positive words, thoughts, and ideas into your mind.
- Affirmations are powerful thoughts deposited into your subconscious.
- Affirmations are the directions that keep your mind on a positive course.
- Affirmations are simple, positive statements, short and to the point.

For example, begin every morning by saying: "Today is a wonderful day." Say it to yourself a few times, then say it out loud. Say it with feeling and conviction. See the wonderful day in your mind's eye.

Of course, saying "Today is a wonderful day" does not change the fact that it is raining and you cannot find your umbrella, that you get stuck in traffic, that your boss yells at you, and that your dinner is burned.

Saying "Today is a wonderful day" instructs your brain not to get stressed over those things. Rain is rain, you can't change that. But you can change how you react to it. Affirmations reprogram your brain, help you change the way you react to potentially stressful situations.

Write those powerful affirmations into your Mental Blueprints. Then, next time it rains you won't react with stress. Instead of having your brain send stressed and diseased messages to your body, you will react by thinking: "Okay, it's raining. I'm not going to get stressed. I'll just put on a raincoat. And if I can't find my raincoat, all right, I'll get wet." It is still raining—but you are not stressed. That's the power of affirmations.

Most of us have programmed our brains with negative thoughts: "My boss is a jerk," "It's a lousy day," "Nobody loves me," "I hate my job." The brain responds to these unhappy thoughts with stress.

Banish those thoughts from your mind. Give your brain healthy, happy thoughts to turn into healthy, happy messages for your body to thrive on.

## AFFIRMATIONS AGAINST PAIN

How do affirmations fit in with chronic pain? Pain is stress. Because pain hurts you respond to it with negative feelings. The brain turns the negative feelings into stressful chemicals, which carry their stressful message to every part of your body.

Pain loves stress. Pain and stress work together, hacking and crushing and squeezing and twisting and jabbing with glee. The pain becomes worse than ever. You respond to the new pain with ever more negative feelings. Your mind is full of these kinds of thoughts:

- "I wish my goddamn arm would fall off!"
- "It's going to be another rotten day!"
- "I can't do anything because my arm hurts so much!"
- "If only my arm didn't hurt so much!"
- "Pain is ruining my life!"

The cycle goes on forever—unless you break it with affirmations. Here are some antipain affirmations I have my patients say:

- I control my life.
- I am in command of my body.
- What I think determines what I feel.
- I think only good thoughts and I feel good!
- Every day I feel better and better.
- I give myself permission to feel great!
- Today is a wonderful day!

Begin with these affirmations. Set aside 10 minutes every morning. Choose a quiet spot where you will not be disturbed. Repeat your affirmations several times silently. Then say them aloud, with strength and belief. Now close your eyes. See your pain. Give it a shape and a size, a texture. For example, see your lower back pain as a baseball. When you say "Every day I feel better and better" see yourself throwing that baseball far away. Watch the baseball as it flies further and further away, getting smaller and smaller, until it has completely vanished. When you say "Today is a wonderful day," picture yourself in your mind's eye. Imagine yourself smiling, happy, and pain-free. See yourself going through the day with a smile on your face.

Repeat your affirmations all during the day: say them in the car, on coffee and lunch breaks; say them to yourself silently at your desk; set aside another 10 minutes every evening for another "Say and See" session.

Fill your brain with your positive affirmations and thoughts. Don't leave any room for negative thoughts. Remember, you are what you think. Negative thoughts and feelings become diseased, painful stress. Positive, happy thoughts translate into health and life.

## THE DUMBEST THING . . . BUT IT WORKS

"I'm not going to say those affirmations. It's silly." That is what Kathy A., a secretary and mother of three told me. She came to see me complaining of lower back pain. I examined her but found nothing wrong with her back. As we talked in my office I could see she was under a great deal of stress at home and at work.

"Why don't you give me some medicine like my other doctors did?" she asked.

"What did they give you?"

"Naprosyn, Empirin with codeine, some others," she answered.

"How's your back?"

"It still hurts."

"The pills didn't work, did they?"

"Give me different ones. Stronger ones," she demanded.

"Listen," I said. "You already have strong drugs. They're not working. I can give you stronger ones but they'll have stronger side effects. Why not try affirmations?" I offered her a paper with several affirmations written on it.

"No." She got up and left, shoving the paper in her .pocket.

I thought I would never see her again. About one month later she called, saying sheepishly, "Dr. Fox, remember me? The one who didn't want to say affirmations. I said them. I thought it was the dumbest thing but my back hurt so much I figured I didn't have anything to lose so I said them. I didn't think they'd work. You know what? They work. I don't get so tense at everything anymore. Getting tense made my back hurt, so learning how to stay calm helped my back. I'm really gung ho on the affirmations now. They sure beat drugs.''

## SAY IT, SEE IT, THEN FEEL IT

After you say it and see it, feel it. Feel it in your heart. Kathy devised clever ways to help herself see and feel herself getting better. She bought a wooden ball and some sandpaper at a lumber store. While she says her affirmations over and over again in the morning and evening she sands down the wooden ball. That helps her feel what she's saying and seeing. Say it and see it—soon you'll feel it.

## TOWERS OF COMPLEX CARBOHYDRATES

Now that the foundation has been laid it is time to build mighty towers and walls of complex carbohydrates. These are the walls that will physically protect you from stress.

What I am going to describe is the dietary philosophy first introduced in my earlier book, *The Beverly Hills* Medical *Diet* (Bantam Books). The dietary descriptions here will be brief. For more information see *The Beverly Hills* Medical *Diet*.

Your food is like your thoughts: Good thoughts = good health, and good foods = good health. The bulk of your diet should consist of complex carbohydrates which are found in vegetables, whole grains, fruits, and legumes (peas, beans, and lentils). Complex carbohydrates are associated with plenty of vitamins, minerals, and fiber; they're delicious, economic, and easy to prepare.

Complex carbohydrates are your body's best source of energy. You can burn fat and protein for energy, but they are second-rate fuels. As protein is burned, nitrogen atoms are released. These can combine with other protein particles to make urea and uric acid. Excess uric acid can cause gout. Burning fat for fuel also leaves your body with the problem of disposing waste products. Complex carbohydrates, on the other hand, are clean burning. Eating lots of fat and/or protein for energy is stressful. Stick with complex carbohydrates. They're your best source of energy.

## ONLY GOOD FOR THE FAT LOBBY

Forty-five percent of the calories the average American eats come from fat. That is well over twice as many calories* from fat as you need: Enough fat to kill you.

We have been trained to eat fat. Cakes, ice cream, pies, candies, desserts, dairy products, junk food, processed foods, and meat are all full of fat. What is wrong with fat? Nothing—if you only eat a little. You need some fat to store energy, cushion organs, carry certain vitamins, and so on. A little is good for you. Too much can kill you—too much *will* kill you.

1. Too much fat means too much weight. Carrying around extra pounds is stressful.
2. Fat helps clog up arteries to the heart, brain, kidney, and other organs. When these arteries close the organs die from lack of nourishment.
3. Cancer, diabetes, and other killer diseases have been strongly linked to excess fat. Directly or indirectly, fat is a killer.

There are lots of people traveling around the country, taking out ads in newspapers and magazines, lobbying in Congress, filling schoolchildren's minds with propaganda, proclaiming that fat is good for you. These people are called the Fat Lobby, and they are funded by the companies that fill supermarkets and restaurants with fatty foods. It's like the wolf giving the farmer a pamphlet explaining why it is a good idea for the farmer to let his chickens and cattle run loose at night. Sure it's a good idea—for the wolf. The Fat Lobby doesn't care if your arteries are filled with fat; they just want their pockets filled with cash.

## PROTEIN MANIA

We are carrying on a love affair with protein in this country. We eat it, drink it, put it in our hair, even rub it on our skin. We

---

*Calories are measures of energy. All the calories you eat come in the form of carbohydrates, protein, or fat. An ounce of fat has just over twice as many calories as an ounce of protein or carbohydrate. Ounce for ounce there is no caloric difference between protein and carbohydrates.

have been taught, incorrectly, that we need to eat a lot of protein. The body uses protein as a structural material, for hormones and other chemicals, and as a fuel. We need some protein, but not nearly as much as we have been led to believe.

When you use protein for fuel there are waste products that have to be dealt with—like the pollutants coming out of the back of our cars. The protein waste products can be just as deadly as the auto emissions if they are not handled properly. You do not have that problem when using complex carbohydrates for fuel because there are no dangerous waste products to dispose of.

We're told that we need protein for strength and endurance. Some years ago a study was conducted to determine which was a better fuel, protein or complex carbohydrates. One group of athletes ate a high-protein diet, the second a diet high in complex carbohydrates, and the third a mixed diet. The three groups were tested for athletic endurance after being on their respective diets for a while. The high complex-carbohydrate diet group lasted almost three times as long as the high-protein group. The mixed-diet group lasted longer than the high-protein group, but not as long as the high complex-carbohydrate group. This study, and others, makes it clear the complex carbohydrates are your best energy source.

Marathon runners know this. Before a race they don't eat steak; they fill up with carbohydrates. Most of us are not athletes, of course. However, we can translate "athletic endurance" into energy for our daily lives. We need complex carbohydrates for energy as much as the athletes do.

## SWEET STRESS

Sugar, along with fat, is the most popular food stressor in this country. It used to be a luxury—now you can hardly keep away from the stuff. Sugar is in everything: canned foods, processed foods, bread, commercial spaghetti, cakes, pies, soda, punch, ice cream, TV dinners, canned fruits, canned vegetables, and almost everything else we eat.

I admit it—sugar tastes good. But how do hypoglycemia, diabetes, and elevated cholesterol taste? Not very good. They don't feel very good, either. Excess consumption of sugar causes diabetes, hypoglycemia, elevated cholesterol, tooth decay, and many other problems. Sugar is stress. (I will talk more about sugar in chapters 5 and 9.)

## SALTY STRESS

To be brief and blunt, eating too much salt can raise your blood pressure. If your blood pressure goes too high your arteries can harden, lose their elasticity, or burst. Too much salt can cause heart disease, stroke, and kidney disease.

How much salt is too much? All the sodium (salt) you need is already in your food, put there by nature. Anything you add and anything the food processors add is dangerous. (I will talk more about salt in chapter 9.)

## DR. FOX'S ANTISTRESS DIET

Here is what my Antistress Diet boils down to:

| | |
|---|---|
| Complex Carbohydrates | Seventy percent of the calories come from complex carbohydrates |
| Protein | Ten percent of the calories come from protein |
| Fat | Twenty percent of the calories come from fat |

Compare that to what you are currently eating, the Standard American Diet (SAD):

| | |
|---|---|
| Carbohydrates | About 35 percent of the calories come from carbohydrates. About 75 percent of these are in the form of refined carbohydrates. |
| Protein | About 20 percent of the calories come from protein |
| Fat | About 45 percent of the calories, and often more, come from fat |

What you get with the SAD is too much fat and protein, but not nearly enough complex carbohydrates. You also get plenty of chemicals, sugar, salt, caffeine, and alcohol, none of which is designed to improve your health.

Notice that Dr. Fox's Antistress Diet contains *complex carbohydrates,* while the SAD has *refined carbohydrates.* What's the difference? It's the difference between health and disease.

Carbohydrates, whether simple or complex, are sugars. Complex carbohydrates are long chains of sugars strung tightly together, found in association with lots of fiber. The long chain-complex carbohydrates found in fruit, vegetables and whole grains are slowly broken apart, sending a little sugar at a time into your bloodstream. Refined carbohydrates are foodstuffs made from white flour and sugar. Refined carbohydrates are quickly broken down inside your body, flooding your bloodstream with a lot of sugar all at once—too much for your body to handle.

Simple carbohydrates are also called simple sugars. Table sugar and the other sugars dumped into your foods are simple sugars. These are the sugars that cause hypoglycemia, diabetes, elevated cholesterol, and other problems.

Complex carbohydrates are also called starches. Starches are great for you, they're very healthy. Unfortunately, many people think that starchy foods (like potatoes and bread) are fattening. That is not true. Potatoes are *not* fattening. The mountains of butter and sour cream you plop on the potatoes *are* fattening. A potato has about as many calories as an apple. Likewise, bread made from complex carbohydrates is *not* fattening. Jelly, jam, and butter *are* fattening. Commercial breads made from white flour (which is not a complex carbohydrate because of the refining process) and filled with simple sugars are junk.

When you are on Dr. Fox's Antistress Diet, most of the carbohydrates you eat are complex, nutritious carbohydrates; less than half the carbohydrates on the SAD are complex. Many of them are in the form of highly refined, simple sugar—a poison.


## DO'S AND DON'TS FOR THE ANTISTRESS DIET

**DO:**

• Eat plenty of complex carbohydrates.
• Eat lots of natural, unprocessed foods.
• Drink plenty of water.

- Eat fresh, lightly cooked vegetables.
- Eat plenty of whole grains (such as rice, barley, oats, millet, and whole wheat).
- Eat a wide variety of fresh, unprocessed foods.
- Eat as close to nature as possible.

**DO NOT:**

- Don't eat junk foods.
- Don't eat processed foods.
- Don't eat fatty foods.
- Don't eat sugar and sugary foods.
- Don't eat salt and salty foods.
- Don't eat processed foods full of chemicals and additives.
- Don't eat a lot of foods containing cholesterol (dairy products, eggs, meat, poultry, fish).
- Don't drink more than an occasional cup of coffee or tea. If you can do without coffee and tea altogether, so much the better.
- Don't have more than an occasional alcoholic drink. If you don't have to, don't drink alcohol at all.

I am not saying you should never eat any fat, salt, or sugar, or never do anything on my Do Not list. You need a little bit of fat, and a little bit of salt or sugar is not going to kill you. But stick with the Do's as much as possible and stay away from the Don'ts. As for cheating, well, you're only hurting yourself.

At the end of this chapter you will find lists of the different foods you should and should not eat on Dr. Fox's Antistress Diet, and some sample recipes to get you started. Before we get there, however, let's take a quick look at a few more important issues.

## DO I NEED SUPPLEMENTARY VITAMINS AND MINERALS?

My patients often ask me whether they need dietary supplements—I tell them that if we lived in an ideal environment, if our food was grown in pure air and nutritious soil, if we ate our food relatively soon after it was picked, if we ate a wide variety of foods, and if we were not so stressed, we probably would not need vitamins and minerals. Unfortunately, we do not live in utopia, so the answer is yes, most of us need vitamin and mineral supplements.

Vitamins are small, organic molecules that help keep the body's enzyme systems running. Without vitamins many of the chemical reactions that take place inside your body would, for all practical purposes, cease; that is why they are called the "spark plugs of life."

Minerals are inorganic elements found in the earth's crust. We need small amounts of many minerals to stay healthy—and to stay alive.

The average person eats three to four pounds of food a day. Only a tiny proportion of that must be in the form of vitamins and minerals to safeguard your health. That doesn't seem like much, but most of us do not have enough of several vitamins and minerals. There are a number of reasons for this sad state of health, including the following:

• Modern growing, processing, and marketing practices give us food that is a nutritional joke, lacking in vitamins and minerals.
• Cooking and freezing destroys vitamins.
• Air and water pollution increase our need for vitamins and minerals.
• Many common drugs interfere with the body's ability to utilize vitamins and minerals.
• We use up vitamins digesting junk foods.
• Stress eats into our nutrient stores.

The list goes on. The basic idea is this: Because of our modern life-style we need more and more vitamins and minerals, but our foods are providing us with less and less vitamins and minerals. We need more but we get less. The result is a nutrient gap. Unless the gap is filled you will be stressed, and stress creates pain and disease.

## ANTIPAIN VITAMINS AND MINERALS

Every individual is unique and nutrient requirements vary from one person to the next. I cannot prescribe vitamins and minerals without first examining a person. This is the nutrient regimen I have most of my patients start with:

**VITAMIN A**—I tell my patients to get their vitamin A from their food. Green and orange vegetables and orange fruits are high in beta carotene, the plant form of vitamin A. The beta carotene you eat is converted by your body into vitamin A. Beta carotene is a better and safer way of getting vitamin A than taking supplements because you cannot overdose on beta carotene; if you have too much, your body will stop converting it to vitamin A. With vitamin A supplements there is the possibility of getting too much vitamin A. I tell my patients to eat two or three whole carrots a day because carrots have 8,000 to 10,000 International Units (IU) of vitamin A (in the form of beta carotene). Three and a half ounces of broccoli have 2,500 IU.

**B VITAMINS**—I suggest my patients take a B-complex vitamin containing 50 mg of the major B vitamins. I have them take one tablet twice a day.

**VITAMIN C**—I suggest my patients take 1,000 mg of time-released vitamin C twice a day.

**VITAMIN D**—As a rule, I do not recommend vitamin D to my patients. In warm or moderate climates (such as that in southern California) you can get all the vitamin D you need from the action of the sunlight on your skin. In addition, foods such as milk have been irradiated to provide vitamin D.

**VITAMIN E**—I recommend my patients start with 200 to 400 mg of D-alpha tocopherol (vitamin E) twice a day.

**MINERALS**—I have my patients begin with a multiple mineral that contains 1/4 of the recommended daily allowance (RDA) for all the minerals, and take four tablets a day. In addition, I often often suggest an extra 100 mg of zinc, 100 mcg (micrograms) of selenium, and 100–200 mcg of chromium.

This is the basic pain supplementation plan. I tailor it to the individual patient's needs, giving more or less of the various nutrients as necessary.

## NATURE'S NUTRITIONAL CORNUCOPIA

For extra strength in their stress-proof castles of pain-free health I have my patients drink aloe vera juice. Aloe vera juice comes from the aloe vera plant. It is a member of the lily family; it's a plant with a long medicinal history. Ancient people did not know why, but they knew that aloe vera was a marvelous health and general tonic. Today we know that stabilized aloe vera juice contains:

| VITAMINS | MINERALS |
|---|---|
| A (beta carotene)* | Calcium |
| $B_1$ (Thiamine) | Chloride |
| $B_2$ (Riboflavin) | Chromium |
| $B_3$ (Niacin) | Copper |
| $B_6$ (Pyridoxine) | Magnesium |
| Folic Acid | Potassium |
| C** | Sodium |
| E*** | Zinc |

*Beta carotene is activated during the stabilization procedure.
**Additional vitamin C is added to the precasting vitamin C during stabilization.
***Vitamin E (alpha tocopherol) is added during the stabilization procedure.

In early 1983 I discovered that aloe vera also contains small amounts of vitamin $B_{12}$. For that story see my article in *Total Health*.[1]

Besides the vitamins and minerals I have listed, aloe vera juice contains amino acids and other nutrients. That's why I call aloe vera nature's nutritional cornucopia. It is chock-full of nutrients that help you strengthen your stress-free castles of health. Aloe vera is like an extra layer of mortar and bricks on your castle's wall, an extra bit of protection for your general health.

Because I have observed that aloe vera juice is such an excellent general tonic and promoter of good health, I have my patients begin by drinking 2 ounces of aloe vera juice with breakfast (mixed with juice). They slowly add more aloe juice, up until bowel tolerance (loose stools). When they reach bowel tolerance I have them drop down to the next lower dosage (or further if necessary). They remain at the dosage just below their bowel tolerance. Here is the plan I start my patients on:

**Day 1:**  2 ounces with breakfast
**Day 4:**  Add 2 ounces with lunch
**Day 7:**  Add 2 ounces with dinner
Patients are now taking 2 ounces three times a day.
They continue on this schedule until:
**Day 15:** Add 2 ounces to the breakfast dose
**Day 18:** Add 2 ounces to the lunch dose
**Day 21:** Add 2 ounces to the dinner dose
They are now taking 4 ounces three times a day.

Four ounces three times a day (with meals) is the basic dosage. If my patients can take more, great. Some report drinking up to 20 ounces a day.

## SURROUND YOUR CASTLE WALLS WITH WATER

Every part of your body, from the largest organ to the smallest cell, needs water. About 60 percent of the average male body and 50 percent of the average female body is composed of water. Every single one of the billions of cells in your body needs enough water inside of it, and enough surrounding it, to carry out its assigned duties.

Every day you lose between a quart and a quart and a half of water in your urine, and up to a quart through your skin (perspiration). You also lose water in the stool and with exhaled breath. If you do not drink enough water to compensate for these loses your body will begin to hoard water, storing it in tissues, especially the tissue around your abdomen.

Drink plenty of water. It helps keep you cool and carries off wastes, among other things. I tell my patients to drink 8 to 10 glasses of water a day. This may seem like a lot of water at first, but you can easily work your way up to this amount in two or three weeks. Just drink a little more every day.

## PA WALKING

Positive Affirmation (PA) Walking is a way of strengthening your body *and* your Mental Blueprints at the same time.

Positive Affirmation Walking is very easy. You just step out your door and start walking. Go out every day and walk as far as you can. Every block repeat an affirmation in your head. If you walk 10 blocks, that's 10 affirmations.

Make it a brisk walk—as brisk as you can. Keep walking farther and faster until you can PA Walk two miles in 30 minutes. When you can PA Walk two miles at this speed every evening, move up to PA Jogging, PA Bicycling, or PA Swimming.

The basic PA idea can be applied to any aerobic exercise. If you are PA Jogging around a track, say an affirmation every time you begin a new lap. When PA Swimming, each new lap is the time for another affirmation. For PA Aerobic Dancing, say an affirmation to yourself every time you switch to a new movement, or every time the music changes.

Which affirmations should you say in your head while PA Exercising? Use modified pain affirmations. Here is a sample based on the affirmation I gave you earlier in this chapter:

I am now in control of my life.
I am in command of my body.
I think only good thoughts and I feel good!
Exercise adds to those good feelings.
Every step (lap) I take makes me stronger and healthier.
I'm thinking and exercising myself into great health!

I PA Jog around the local high-school track every morning. I say two affirmations a lap. I usually run about 12 laps (three miles), so I say 24 affirmations. I have four different PA Jogging affirmations. During the course of my morning PA Jog I say each one six times. Strengthening both body and Mental Blueprints is a great way to start the day!

With PA Walking, PA Jogging, PA Aerobic Dancing, or any aerobic exercise, the goal is to raise your heart rate (the number of beats per minute) to between 70 and 80 percent of its maximal rate, and keep it there for 20 to 30 minutes.

To find your "target zone" (70–80% of maximal rate) locate

your age along the bottom axis of this chart. Follow your age line into the shaded area.

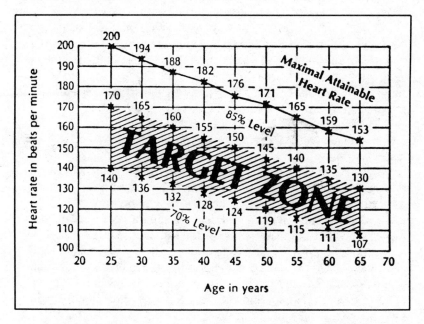

When you PA exercise wear a watch with a second hand so you can check your heart rate. Stop every 15 minutes to check your pulse. Do this by pressing your index and middle fingers on your wrist (outside corner), temples, or the base of your neck. Count the number of beats you feel for 6 seconds, multiply this number by 10 to get your heart rate per minute. Compare your heart rate to the chart above. If you are in your target zone, great! If not, adjust your speed (faster or slower) and keep going.

PA Walking, PA Jogging, PA Swimming, PA Aerobic Dancing, PA Bicycling, any exercise that gets your heart beating in its target zone for 20 to 30 minutes is great. And adding Positive Affirmations makes it a total *body and mind* workout!

CAUTION: *If you are over age 30, or if you have any history or indications of heart or respiratory trouble, see your physician before you begin, or change, an exercise program. If you have any difficulties related to exercising see your physician immediately.*

## TO EAT OR NOT TO EAT—LISTS

Now that the basics of Dr. Fox's Antistress Diet have been covered, let's get down to specifics: What can you eat?

This is what you eat on my Antistress Diet: Fresh fruits, fresh vegetables, whole grains, and legumes (peas, beans, lentils), and small amounts of low-fat fish, poultry, and dairy products (and small amounts of red meat if desired). The Antistress Diet is rich in complex carbohydrates, vitamins, minerals, fiber, and all the other nutrients you need to build the best of health.

The best way to eat vegetables is lightly steamed or cooked. Processing, storing, freezing, and cooking tend to destroy or leach out many of the nutrients in vegetables. I suggest to my patients that they eat their vegetables lightly steamed because that way they are warm, crunchy, and full of nutrition.

Raw vegetables are also excellent; easy to prepare (wash and peel), crunchy, and nutritious. Eat them separately or cut up and mix in a bowl with raisins, nuts, parmesan cheese, etc.

Whole grains are tasty, nutritious, and easy to prepare. You cook them as you would cook rice. Some take longer to cook than rice does, some take less time. I like to mix them, cook seven or eight of them in one pot and eat them together. You can throw in chopped vegetables and/or nuts if you like.

## FOODS FOR VITAMINS

Here are lists of foods which contain good amounts of vitamins. Foods in parentheses are high in fat or cholesterol: Use these foods sparingly.

VITAMIN A

| | | |
|---|---|---|
| red chili peppers | swiss chard | endive |
| dandelion greens | chives | apricots |
| carrots | butternut squash | broccoli |
| collard, kale | watercress | green onions |
| sweet potatoes | mangos | romaine |
| parsley | sweet red pepper | papayas |
| spinach | winter squash | nectarines |
| turnip, mustard greens | cantaloupe | |

VITAMIN B₁ (Thiamine)

| | | |
|---|---|---|
| pinto and red beans | lima beans, dry | whole-grain rice |
| split peas | (hazelnuts) | (walnuts) |
| millet | wild rice | garbanzos |
| navy beans | whole grain rye | garlic |
| buckwheat | whole grain cornmeal | (almonds) |
| whole grain oats | lentils | |
| whole grain wheat | green peas | |

VITAMIN B₂ (Riboflavin)

| | | |
|---|---|---|
| wild rice | parsley | whole-grain rye |
| mushrooms | broccoli | pinto and red beans |
| millet | chicken/turkey | black-eyed peas |
| hot red peppers | (salmon) | okra |
| collards | navy beans | (sesame seeds) |
| split peas | beet and mustard greens | (pine nuts) |
| kale | lentils | |

VITAMIN B₃ (Niacin)

| | | |
|---|---|---|
| turkey, white meat | whole-grain rice | barley |
| chicken, white meat | (pine nuts) | (almonds) |
| brook trout | buckwheat | (shrimp) |
| halibut | red chili peppers | haddock |
| (salmon) | whole-grain wheat | split peas |
| (sesame seeds) | mushrooms | |

VITAMIN B₅ (Pantothenic Acid)
Pantothenic acid is so named because it is found everywhere (pan = all). The highest amounts of B₅ are found in:

whole grain cereals
legumes (peas, beans, lentils)
fish
(meat)

## VITAMIN B$_6$ (Pyridoxine)

tuna
(walnuts)
(salmon)
brook trout
lentils
lima beans, dry
buckwheat
black-eyed peas
navy beans
whole-grain rice
(hazelnuts)
garbanzos

pinto beans
bananas
albacore
halibut
(avocados)
whole-grain wheat
chestnuts
kale
whole-grain rye
spinach
turnip greens
sweet red pepper

potatoes
sardines
brussels sprouts
perch
cod
barley
sweet potatoes
cauliflower
popcorn
red cabbage
leeks

## VITAMIN B$_{12}$

sardines
brook trout
(salmon)
tuna
haddock

flounder
scallops
cottage cheese, low fat
halibut
perch

## VITAMIN C

red chili peppers
guavas
red sweet peppers
kale
parsley
collards
turnip greens
green sweet peppers
broccoli
brussels sprouts
mustard greens
cauliflower
persimmons
red cabbage
strawberries
papayas

spinach
oranges
cabbage
lemons
grapefruit
turnips
mangoes
watercress
asparagus
cantalope
swiss chard
green onions
okra
tangerines
New Zealand spinach
(oysters)

lima beans
black-eyed peas
green peas
radishes
raspberries
chinese cabbage
yellow summer squash
honeydew melon
tomatoes

## VITAMIN E

green leafy vegetables          (wheat-germ oil)
milk                            (peanut oil)
(lean meats)

# FOODS FOR MINERALS

(Foods in parentheses are also high in fat and/or cholesterol.)

## CALCIUM

| | | |
|---|---|---|
| collard, turnip greens | romaine lettuce | onions |
| (almonds) | rutabaga | lemons |
| parsley | green beans | green peas |
| corn tortillas, lime added | globe artichokes | cauliflower |
| dandelion greens | dry beans | lentils |
| watercress | cabbage | cherries |
| buttermilk | sprouts | asparagus |
| yogurt | whole grain wheat | winter squash |
| beet greens | oranges | strawberries |
| buckwheat | celery | millet |
| (sesame seeds) | whole grain rice | pineapple |
| broccoli | carrots | grapes |
| (walnuts) | barley | beets |
| cottage cheese, low fat | sweet potatoes | cantaloupe |
| spinach | garlic | |
| milk, non-fat or skim | summer squash | |

## IRON

| | |
|---|---|
| millet | whole-grain wheat |
| parsley | beet greens |
| kidney beans | swiss chard |
| dried split peas | dandelion greens |
| (oysters) | (walnuts) |
| (almonds) | spinach |
| (hazelnuts) | (sesame seeds) |
| whole-grain oats | (pecans) |
| sardines | lentils |
| Jerusalem artichokes | |

## MAGNESIUM

| | | |
|---|---|---|
| (almonds) | dry beans | green peppers |
| buckwheat | barley | winter squash |
| (filbert nuts) | dandelion greens | cantaloupe |
| millet | garlic | eggplant |
| whole-grain wheat | fresh green peas | tomato |
| (pecans) | potato with skin | cabbage |
| (walnuts) | banana | grapes |
| whole-grain rye | sweet potatoes | skim milk |
| beet greens | blackberries | pineapple |
| spinach | beets | mushrooms |
| whole-grain rice | broccoli | onions |
| swiss chard | cauliflower | oranges |
| collard greens | carrots | plums |
| corn | celery | apples |
| (avocado) | asparagus | |
| parsley | turkey/chicken | |

## MANGANESE

| | | |
|---|---|---|
| cloves | whole-grain wheat | buckwheat |
| wheat bran | ginger | (peanuts) |
| rice bran | spinach | blueberries |
| oat bran | whole-grain rice | pineapple |
| (walnuts) | whole-grain oats | |

## SELENIUM

| | | |
|---|---|---|
| apple cider vinegar | turnips | onions |
| scallops | garlic | carrots |
| barley | barley | cabbage |
| whole-grain wheat | mushrooms | oranges |
| (shrimp) | turkey/chicken | |
| red swiss chard | radishes | |
| whole-grain oats | (pecans) | |
| (king crab) | (hazelnuts) | |
| skim milk | (almonds) | |
| cod | green beans | |
| whole-grain rice | kidney beans | |

ZINC

| | |
|---|---|
| ginger root | buckwheat |
| (pecans) | (hazel nuts) |
| split peas | (clams) |
| whole-grain wheat | tuna |
| whole-grain rye | haddock |
| whole-grain oats | green peas |
| lima beans | turnips |
| (almonds) | black pepper, paprika |
| (walnuts) | dry mustard, chili powder |
| sardines | thyme and cinnamon have |
| turkey/chicken | appreciable amounts of zinc |

As you look over these lists of foods high in vitamins and minerals, you'll notice that they are, for the most part, vegetables, fruits, whole grains, nuts, seeds, and fish—exactly the kinds of foods you're eating on the Antistress Diet. These foods are also high in fiber, with just the right amounts of sodium and natural sugar (simple carbohydrates).

The Antistress Diet is very simple. There are no formulas to worry about, you don't have to eat certain foods on specific days. Just eat a wide variety of fresh vegetables and fruits, whole grains, nuts, seeds, and small amounts of low-fat fish, poultry, and dairy products (and small amounts of lean meat if desired).

## SAMPLE RECIPES FOR THE ANTISTRESS DIET

Here are a few recipes to give you some ideas of what can be done with all those vegetables, fruits, whole grains, nuts, and seeds.

### *Herbal Dressing*

1 large clove garlic, crushed
2 teaspoons chopped chives or green onion tops
3/4 teaspoon dill weed
1/2 teaspoon each dry mustard and paprika
1/4 teaspoon each tarragon and chervil
1 tablespoon mild vinegar
1 cup low-fat yogurt
1/2 cup buttermilk

Place garlic, chives, seasoning and vinegar in blender and blend at low speeds. Then add yogurt and buttermilk and blend thoroughly. Store in tightly covered jar in refrigerator. Will keep about 1 week.

*Makes about 2 cups*

### *Apple Bran Muffins*

1 cup grated raw apples, packed
3/4 cup bran or 1/2 cup wheat germ and 1/2 cup bran
3/4 cup old-fashioned rolled oats
1/4 teaspoon white pepper, if desired
1/2 cup chopped dates simmered in small amount of
    water to soften
2 tablespoons raw cashews plus 1/4 cup orange juice
    concentrate blended with the dates until smooth

Combine all ingredients in large mixing bowl and let stand 5–10 minutes. Spray muffin pans and pack mixture into them to about 1 inch thickness. Bake at 375°F. for approximately 30 minutes or until lightly browned.

*Makes 1 dozen muffins*

### Vegetable Barley Soup

Dry-sauté (cook in heavy skillet, without fat or oil, over low heat, keep covered):

1 onion, diced
1 clove garlic
1 green pepper, diced

When tender add to soup pot with:

6 cups water, boiling
4 tomatoes, chopped
1/2 cup barley
1 teaspoon Tamari soy sauce (reduced salt type)
1 teaspoon dried basil
1 teaspoon dried oregano
1/8 teaspoon cayenne

When barley is almost tender (about 45 minutes) add:

2 cups broccoli, finely chopped
3 carrots, diced
1 cup celery, diced

Cook till the vegetables are tender/crisp.

*Serves 4–6*

### Cucumbers with Yogurt

2 cups cucumbers, thinly sliced
2 cups low-fat yogurt (skim-milk yogurt preferably)
1 clove garlic, pressed
1 tablespoon vinegar
1/2 teaspoon dill
2 tablespoons finely chopped scallion
1 tablespoon fresh mint

Mix together and marinate for 1 hour. Serve on bed of romaine lettuce leaves. Garnish with 1 cup seedless green grapes when available.

*Serves 2–4*

## *Herbal Omelet*

6 egg whites
¼ teaspoon white pepper
2 tablespoons fresh snipped parsley
1 tablespoon fresh snipped tarragon leaves
1 tablespoon fresh snipped marjoram leaves
½ tablespoon fresh snipped thyme leaves
1 tablespoon finely chopped shallots

If you use dry herbs, halve the quantity.

Combine egg whites, pepper, and 1 tablespoon cold water in bowl. Beat with rotary beater until just combined, not frothy. Mix in all other ingredients and mix well with spatula. Spray non-aluminum fry pan with Pam and heat slowly.

Turn egg mixture into skillet and cook slowly over medium heat. Be sure to lift edges of omelet so uncooked portion can run under cooked part of omelet.

When omelet is dry on top and slightly golden brown on bottom, fold it over to edge of pan and carefully slip out onto serving dish.

*Serves 2*

## *Rice Casserole with Tuna*

2 seven-ounce cans water-packed Albacore tuna fish
3 cups cooked brown rice
1 cup sliced celery
½ cup chopped onions
1 cucumber that has been liquified in blender
⅓ cup nonfat milk
1 cup grated low-salt low-fat cheese (such as farmers
    or pot cheese)

Combine tuna, rice, celery, and onions, and set aside. Blend the milk and cheese, mix with the cucumber, and heat slowly in a nonaluminum pot. Add tuna, rice, celery, and onions together with your favorite seasonings and turn into a Pam-sprayed casserole (2 quart). Bake at 375°F for 20 minutes or until hot and bubbly.

*Serves 6*

## *Meatless Burger*

1 cup cooked drained barley, rice, or cracked wheat
1 cup slightly crushed cooked chickpeas, navy beans,
    or pinto beans
1/3 cup quick cooking oatmeal (raw)
1 tablespoon paprika
1/4 tablespoon reduced salt soy sauce
Dash or two of chili powder
Other spices to taste

In a blender or food processor finely chop

2 egg whites
1 small stalk celery
1/2 small onion
1 scallion
1 clove garlic
1 large tomato

Mix together all ingredients and blend well. Shape into patties or balls.

Heat small amount of water in nonaluminum fry pan and brown patties over medium heat 3–5 minutes on each side or until lightly browned.

*Makes 6 burgers*

### Fish Baked in Yogurt

½ cup yogurt
1 teaspoon onion powder
1 teaspoon dill weed
Dash pepper or paprika

Spread on fish steaks, then bake or broil until done. Do not turn.

### Red Snapper in Cider

2 whole red snappers (about 3 pounds) or 2 pounds
    fillets
10 cups water
2 cups hard cider
½ cup tarragon vinegar
2 onions, sliced
2 carrots, sliced
1 bouquet garni
Pinch mace
Lemon slices for garnish

Set fish aside. Bring other ingredients gently to a boil and simmer 45 minutes in poaching pan. Add fish and poach gently 15 minutes per pound of fish if whole; 15 minutes total cooking time if fish is filleted. May be served hot or cold, garnished with lemon slices and sprigs of fresh dill if available.

*Serves 4*

### Tangy Tuna

Mix one small can drained water-packed tuna (6½ or 7 oz) with ¼ cup chopped celery, 1 tablespoon minced onion, ¼ cup grated carrots. Stir in enough low-fat yogurt to make a thick mixture. Serve on romaine leaves, with a chunk of hoop cheese and a ripe pear.

*Serves 2 for lunch*

### Baked Onions and Millet

2 onions, chopped
1 cup millet
½ teaspoon coriander
½ teaspoon cinnamon
2 cloves garlic, pressed or minced
3 cups water or vegetable water, boiling
¼ cup raisins
A dash of cayenne

Dry-sauté onions. Add to other ingredients, bake 60 minutes at 350°F.

*Serves 1 or 2*

### Split-Pea Stew

1½ cups split peas
4 cups water
1 medium onion, chopped
½ teaspoon garlic (fresh or powder)
½ cup chopped celery
2 medium carrots, sliced
2 medium potatoes, diced
1 teaspoon white pepper

Put split peas, water, onion, garlic, and celery in a large nonaluminum soup pot, bring to a boil and then simmer for 15 minutes. Add carrots, potatoes, and pepper, continue simmering until all ingredients are tender. Add your favorite seasonings.

*Serve 4–6*

## *Lima-and-Rice Burgers*

1½ cups cooked brown rice
1½ cups cooked limas
¾ cup water
¼ tablespoon garlic, fresh or powder
white pepper to taste
Other seasonings as desired

Blend limas in liquid until fine. Add other ingredients and mix well. Drop from spoon or scoop into baking dish (sprayed with Pam). Bake at 350–375°F for about 30 minutes or until lightly browned.

*Should make about 6–8 burgers.*


## *Sautéing Vegetables Without Fat (or Oil)*

Place a little water in bottom of skillet. Add chopped vegetables and cook on low or medium heat until tender. Stir as needed. A little extra water may be added if vegetables become too dry during cooking process.

## *Corn Chowder*

6 cups water
1 teaspoon white pepper
3 cups fresh stewed tomatoes
1 cup diced celery
1 cup diced potatoes
½ cup diced onion
2 cups whole-kernel corn

Combine all ingredients and cook in a nonaluminum pot until vegetables are tender.
In a Crockpot—combine ingredients and cook on low 6–8 hours or on high 3–4 hours.

*Serves 4–6*

## Vegetable Loaf

1 cup fresh string beans (cooked for 3 min. and sliced
    into 1/2-inch strips)
1 cup fresh peas
2 cups grated carrots
2 cups chopped celery
1 cup ground raw sunflower seeds
1/2 cup shredded cabbage or spinach
1 tablespoon lemon juice
1 tablespoon minced onion
1/8 teaspoon garlic (fresh or powdered)
1 teaspoon dry ground bell pepper
1 teaspoon fresh chopped parsley

Mix together all ingredients. Use liquid from cooked string
beans and apple juice concentrate to make 1 1/2 cups liquid, and
mix with vegetables and all other ingredients; press into glass loaf
pan that has been sprayed with Pam.

Bake at 350°F. 20–30 minutes until vegetables are tender.

*Serves 4*

## Kasha Salad

1 cup toasted buckwheat
2 cups boiling water

Pour boiling water over buckwheat, cover, let stand for 20
minutes. Cool. Add:

1/2 onion, finely chopped
2 stalks celery, chopped
1 cucumber, chopped
1 green or red bell pepper, chopped
1 carrot, grated
4–5 radishes, sliced
1 cup cooked green beans
1/2 cup parsley, minced

DRESSING:

    1/2 cup yogurt
    1/4 cup cider or wine vinegar (if desired)
    1/2 teaspoon Tamari soy sauce

*Serves 4*

## Sprout Salad

    1 pound bean and alfalfa sprouts
    1 stalk chopped celery
    1 red apple, unpeeled and chopped
    2 green onions, chopped
    1 handful nuts and raisins

Combine ingredients. Serve with Herbal Dressing (see p. 56).

*Serves 4*

## Fish–Rice Salad

    3 cups cooked brown rice, chilled
    1/2 cup minced celery
    1/2 cup minced green onion
    1/2–1 cup chopped tomato
    2 tablespoons minced parsley
    1–1 1/2 teaspoons dried basil or tarragon
    1 1/2–2 cups cooked fish, chilled and flaked
    4 tablespoons vinegar
    1/2 teaspoon vinegar
    1/2 teaspoon pepper
    1 tablespoon Dijon-style mustard

Serve on shredded romaine. Garnish with tomato wedges.

*Serves 4*

## *Salad in a Sandwich*

Heat pita or Bible bread. When heated, open bread and fill with:

cooked pinto or kidney beans, chili, sprouts, onions, tomatoes, dash of picante sauce (buy at any market), sliced zucchini, grated carrots, grated cabbage

*Makes 1 sandwich*

## *Golden Sauce for Vegetables*

Blend together until smooth:

3/4 cooked potato
1 medium cooked carrot
1 1/3 cups water
2 tablespoons cashews
1 tablespoon lemon juice
garlic and white pepper to taste

Heat and serve over vegetables.

*Makes about 1 cup*

These are just a few recipes to get you started. For a more complete selection of recipes see *The Beverly Hills* Medical *Diet.*

You do not have to be fancy to be healthy. I love to chop up a bunch of vegetables, especially cabbage, and throw it in the lentil stew we often eat. It's simple, nutritious, and tasty, too.

## "SHE WALKED"

One of my early chronic pain/DLPA cases involved an elderly woman named Maxine N. She was a very frail-looking but very lively widow and grandmother. She must have been very strong because she had endured 20 years of severe chronic lower back pain. She described her pain as "burning hot coals sewn into my back."

"How did you manage?" I asked her.

"I refused to give in to the pain. I never let my pain get me down. I never complained. I raised my two youngest after the pain started," she stated proudly. But three years ago her husband had died. Her children were grown, out of the house, some lived in distant cities. Without her husband, with her family dispersed, she found it harder and harder to resist and ignore her pain. Although too proud to complain, it was clear her pain was giving her a great deal of trouble. It was difficult for her to walk, bend over, or twist. This once active woman was reduced to sitting in a chair and knitting most of the day.

Maxine's youngest daughter brought her to see me. She explained that her mother had already been to several doctors and pain clinics.

"Dr. Fox, Mom doesn't complain, but *I* can't stand seeing her sit in the chair all day, *I* can't stand her having to take those pills that don't work, and *I* couldn't stand her two surgeries that didn't do much either. If you can't help her tell me now. I don't want her going through any more useless junk that doesn't help!"

I examined Maxine, studied her records, and performed various tests, including a study of her diet and life-style. Like the other doctors I found no physical problem. I put her on Dr. Fox's DLPA Antipain Program with special emphasis on her Mental Blueprints. She was a strong woman who believed in herself. Believing in her health would help her quite a bit, I felt.

Nothing happened for two weeks. Her daughter told me that Maxine was faithfully sticking to the Antipain Plan, eating what I told her to, saying her affirmations, and taking the DLPA.

A week after that her daughter excitedly phoned me to say: "Dr. Fox! Mom walked half a mile to the grocery store then all the way back carrying a shopping bag!" Within three weeks about 80 percent of Maxine's pain was gone and she was back to her old, lively self. She challenged me to a long distance PA jogging race. I declined—she would have beaten me.

## MAKE SURE YOUR DLPA IS THE "REAL THING"

I tell my patients to make sure they are getting the real thing when they purchase DLPA. I have had bad experiences using generic brands that were ineffective.

Some companies have apparently been manufacturing tablets or capsules with "feed grade" DL-phenylalanine. Feed grade amino acids are meant for animal, not human consumption. Some companies seem to be selling products diluted with excessive LPA, or other amino acids falsely labeled as DLPA. Some of my patients have complained that "DLPA" did not help them. When I put them on a certified brand of DLPA they enjoyed excellent results.

Certified DLPA manufactured by reputable firms is pure, not diluted with inappropriate fillers or other amino acids. DL-phenylalanine made by conscientious companies will be guaranteed to dissolve in seven minutes in the stomach, and therefore have a reliable "bioavailability." (I have used brands of DLPA that contain proper amounts of the amino acid but do not dissolve easily and are therefore ineffective.)

Be aware of what you are buying—make sure you are getting true DLPA. Deal with reputable companies. Check with your health food store.

## WRAP-UP

Well, there you have Dr. Fox's DLPA Antipain Plan. I cannot emphasize strongly enough that every element, every part of the plan, is important.

The diet, vitamins, and minerals, and aloe vera juice help build up your general physical health and resistance to disease.

Mental Blueprints, affirmations, and "saying it and seeing it" drive the negative, stressful thoughts from your mind, and replace them with positive health-giving thoughts.

Positive Affirmation walking, or other aerobic exercises add to your general health and well-being, especially the health of your heart.

DL-phenylalanine zeros in on chronic pain.

Dr. Fox's DLPA Antipain Plan is a package plan. I tell my patients not to pick and choose the parts they like best—stick with the entire plan.

## DO NOT SELF-MEDICATE!

One last, very important warning: Do not self-medicate.

*Do not throw away the medicine(s) your doctor has prescribed for you. Do not alter the dosage or stop taking the medicine(s). Discuss DLPA and Dr. Fox's DLPA Program with your physician. A trained professional, your physician will be able to guide you through the intricacies of the human body and mind. The nice thing about DLPA is that it does not interfere with other medication. You and your doctor can try DLPA without stopping your other medications. My experience with my patients has been that with DLPA I can carefully reduce my patient's other medicines and eventually eliminate them.*

# 4

# DEPRESSION: THE MENTAL CRIPPLER

*If there be a hell upon earth, it is to be found in a melancholy man's heart.*

ROBERT BURTON,
*The Anatomy of Melancholy*

As if chronic pain were not enough, mankind has also been plagued by depression, pain's psychic partner. What happens when depression, like cancer, sets in to strangle your happiness? You can lose your appetite, your sexual drive, and your ability to experience pleasure. In exchange, you receive a sense of worthlessness and feelings of unhappiness. You may be plagued by unrealistic and negative self-evaluations, disturbed sleep patterns, constipation, impotence or frigidity, poor memory and other emotional and physical problems. A 55-year-old man describes his depression:

"Nothing is interesting anymore, nothing is worth the effort. I can't make myself care or give a damn about anything anymore. My family, my daughter. I wish I could care again. I can barely work up enough energy to get out of bed in the morning."

An account executive for a major advertising firm, this man's depression was threatening his livelihood. Projecting energy and enthusiasm was an important part of his job.

Various doctors had treated his clinical depression for several years, to no avail. Some of the standard antidepressant drugs helped a bit, but left him feeling "dumb and slow" and with other side effects.

Like so many millions of Americans, this man suffers from a type of depression known as "endogenous depression," so named because it comes from within the brain, seemingly according to its own schedule. Unlike "reactive depression," which can be linked to a triggering event such as loss of a job or death of a loved one, endogenous depression seems to occur for no discernable reason.

## DOUBLE-EDGED SWORD

Chronic pain and depression are especially dangerous when they act together. Pain can cause depression, then the depression fuels the pain. The worst cases involve people with cancer pain, arthritis, lower back pain, and migraines. The victims become depressed because they cannot understand or cope with their pain. As their depression grows they often lose their desire to fight back and get well. General health begins to fail as patients fall into a vicious cycle of pain and depression, more pain and more depression.

Modern medical science does not understand the causes of endogenous depression, but current research into brain chemistry has provided some exciting leads.

## IS DEPRESSION ALL IN YOUR HEAD?

Yes—but not in the way you think. When I say that the depression was all in the heads of the thousands of depressed patients I have seen, I do not mean that they were crazy. What I mean is this: There are many chemical messengers in your brain. These messengers (neurotransmitters) carry information from one nerve cell (neuron) to another. Some of these neurotransmitters can increase brain activity and improve your mood. But if the brain levels of certain key neurotransmitters drop below critical levels you can become depressed. You do not know why you are depressed, it doesn't seem to make any sense to you. Nevertheless, you are depressed.

This is the endogenous depression that mentally cripples many millions of Americans. This is the type of depression that can come from nowhere and linger for years. And it is the kind of depression DLPA is most effective at treating.

## STANDARD TREATMENTS

Most of the standard drug therapies for depression are concerned with manipulating a brain neurotransmitter called norepinephrine (NE). Scientists found that you could make an animal more physically active by injecting NE into its brain. In other words, NE is a brain stimulant. Great, they thought: If we could get more NE into the brains of depressed people it might relieve their symptoms. Injecting NE directly into people's brains was obviously impractical, so researchers looked for drugs that would indirectly raise brain NE levels.

The tricyclics and the monoamine oxidase inhibitors are two major classes of antidepressant drugs. Both of these types of drugs raise brain NE levels. The tricyclics, named for their three-ringed chemical structure, are the most widely prescribed antidepressants. The monoamine oxidase inhibitors are so named because they retard (inhibit) the breakdown (oxidation) of monoamines. Norepinephrine is one of the monoamines which is protected by the monoamine oxidase inhibitor drugs.

The tricyclics have been involved in hundreds of clinical studies. Surprisingly, in only 60 percent of these tests have the tricyclics shown themselves to be significantly more effective than placebo. Indeed, one authority[1] has argued that tricyclics may be only 10 to 20 percent more effective than placebos.

## THE SIDE EFFECTS FROM STANDARD TREATMENTS

Unfortunately, when you take any of the prescription antidepressant drugs you run the risk of serious side effects. Many times psychiatrists have asked me to examine their depressed patients because they wanted me to make sure their antidepressant medication was not seriously harming them. If the patient has been on tricyclics, I pay special attention to the health of their heart. And the monoamine oxidase inhibitors are known for their very toxic effects on the liver. Here is a brief listing of possible adverse reactions to a few antidepressant drugs, taken from the 1983 edition of the *Physician's Desk Reference:*

AMITRIPTYLINE
Trade name: Elavil
Elavil may cause high blood pressure, irregular heart rhythms, heart block, stroke, hallucinations, confusion, tremors, blurred vision, nausea, weakness, testicular swelling in males, and other problems.

IMIPRAMINE
Trade name: Tofranil—the original tricyclic
Tofranil may cause high blood pressure, low blood pressure, heart block, stroke, irregular heart rhythms, anxiety, delusions, numbness, insomnia, seizures, nausea, vomiting, abdominal cramps, impotence, altered liver function, and other problems.

TRANYLCYPROMINE SULFATE
Trade name: Parnate—a monoamine oxidase inhibitor
Possible side effects include anxiety, weakness, dizziness, nausea, abdominal pain, anorexia, chills, blurred vision, impotence, and other problems.

ISOCARBOXAZID
Trade name: Marplan—a monoamine oxidase inhibitor
Problems include dizziness, constipation, headache, postural hypotension, tremors, confusion, weakness, and other problems.

And when you are on the monoamine oxidase inhibitors you have to be very careful about what you eat. You have to watch out for foods containing tryamine, such as aged cheeses, wine, beer, pickled herring, yogurt, liver, and yeast extract. Do you know how many foods have yeast in them? You must also avoid excessive amounts of caffeine and chocolate.

One patient I treated, a 55-year-old housewife, was being given Nardil by her psychiatrist to treat her depression. Nardil is a monoamine oxidase inhibitor. She did not know she shouldn't drink wine while on Nardil. So she drank wine, got dizzy and weak, and was taken to an emergency room. At the emergency room they found that her blood pressure was elevated. The next day her entire body was covered with a gooseflesh-like rash that lingered for three weeks.

Are the benefits worth the possible side effects? For some people they are. These drugs have helped many depressed people with a minimum of side effects. Then again, I have seen many patients who were adversely affected by these drugs.

How about DL-phenylalanine (DLPA)? Is it safer than the antidepressant drugs? DL-phenylalanine is a nutrient your body knows how to deal with while drugs are foreign substances your body is unfamilar with and does not know how to handle. Here is a graph comparing the toxicity of DLPA to some common antidepressant drugs:

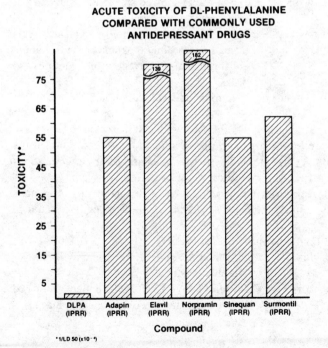

ACUTE TOXICITY OF DL-PHENYLALANINE
COMPARED WITH COMMONLY USED
ANTIDEPRESSANT DRUGS

*1/LD 50 (x10⁻⁹)

As you can see, DLPA barely makes it onto the toxicity chart. You would have to take an incredible amount of DLPA before you could suffer a toxic reaction.

## DLPA VERSUS DEPRESSION

Let's look at some of the scientific research which indicates that DLPA is a safe, effective antidepressant. Here are the results of the first phenylalanine/depression study,[2] conducted by Dr. Yaryura-Tobias at the North Nassau Mental Health Center in New York.

**15 Endogenous Depression Patients**

SYMPTOMS: Symptoms included early morning depression, irregular sleep patterns, lack of drive, feelings of hopelessness and helplessness.

CONDITIONS: Either D-phenylalanine or DL-phenylalanine were given twice daily.

RESULTS: Ten of the 15 showed substantial reduction of symptoms within five days.

COMMENTS: These 10 patients required no further treatment. For the other 5 patients, phenylalanine enhanced the effectiveness of their tricyclic drugs.

SIDE EFFECTS: "No toxic effects" were noted.

In this study DLPA showed itself to be as effective as antidepressant drugs *without serious side effects*. And for the five patients PA did not help, it *worked with their other medication,* making their other medication more effective.

More encouraging results were reported in a second study published in *Arzneimittel Forschung,*[3] a European journal.

**23 Endogenous Depression Patients**

CONDITIONS: Patients were given either D-phenylalanine or DL-phenylalanine.

RESULTS: Within 13 days 17 of the 23 patients returned to a normal state ("complete euthymia").

COMMENTS:    These 17 people had not been helped by previous drug therapy.

SIDE EFFECTS:    No adverse reactions were noted.

Seventeen of 23 is pretty impressive, especially considering that previous antidepressant drugs had not helped them.

More sophisticated studies conducted by Dr. Helmut Beckmann at the Psychiatric Hospital of the University of Munich, West Germany, followed these preliminary reports. Here are the results of Dr. Beckmann's open study[4].

**20 Depressed Patients**

CONDITIONS:    The patients suffered from various kinds of depression.

RESULTS:    Complete to moderate reduction of symptoms for 80 percent of the patients.

COMMENTS:    DLPA showed significant antidepressant properties.

SIDE EFFECTS:    No adverse side effects.

To make sure the DLPA was not harming the patients Dr. Beckmann monitored their brain waves (EEG), heart beat (EKG), and other vital signs. DL-phenylalanine did not have an adverse effect on any of these important indicators. And just as in the previous study, the patients who were helped by DLPA had not been helped by previous treatment with antidepressant drugs.

## OVER 90 PERCENT MAY RESPOND

In 1978 Dr. Heller[5] reported the results of the largest phenylalanine/depression study to date. Over 400 patients suffering from various kinds of depression were involved. Every five days the patients were evaluated by a team of psychiatrists. Physical examinations were given every week. Numerous methods were used to gauge the patient's depression before and during the study. Here are the results for the 370 endogenous depression patients:

| Diagnosis at Beginning of Study | Diagnosis on Day 15 of Study | | | Diagnosis on Day 60 of Study | | |
|---|---|---|---|---|---|---|
| | NAS | I | NI | NAS | I | NI |
| Endogenous Depression | 73% | 23% | 4% | 80% | 15% | 5% |

Key: NAS = Normal Affective State, all depressive symptoms gone.
    I = Improvement, most symptoms relieved
    NI = No Improvement

In 80 percent of the patients all the depressive symptoms cleared up and they regained their ability to work. Another 15 percent enjoyed relief from most of their symptoms. (I have not included the results for patients suffering from other kinds of depression, such as age-related depression. All categories responded well.)

## D-PHENYLALANINE VERSUS A TRICYCLIC: HEAD TO HEAD

In a separate double-blind study,[6] Dr. Heller compared D-phenylalanine to imipramine (trade name Tofranil). Imipramine is the most commonly prescribed tricyclic antidepressant. Sixty patients were divided evenly into two groups. For 15 days one group was given D-phenylalanine, the other imipramine. Then, for 5 days, both groups were given a placebo. For the remaining 10 days each group received their original medication. Here are the results:

| | Percent of Patients Showing Improvement* | | |
|---|---|---|---|
| | After 15 days | 5-Day Placebo Period | After 30 Days |
| D-phenylalanine Group | 83% | 12% | 83% |
| Imipramine Group | 57% | 9% | 73% |

*Includes patients showing improvement (I) and those reaching a normal affective state (NAS).

This study shows that D-phenylalanine is at least as effective as imipramine, and without the side effects.

DL-phenylalanine was again compared to imipramine in a 1979 double-blind study[7] conducted by Helmut Beckmann et al. The patients' depression was assessed using several different systems. Every day their blood pressure, brain waves, pulse rates, and body temperature were checked to see if there were any adverse effects.

The results? DL-phenylalanine was found to be equally effective in treating depression as imipramine was—without imipramine's side effects.

## "A NEW WOMAN"

We've looked at the studies. Now let's see how DLPA has helped some of my patients.

Marie F. is a 60-year-old widow. Her psychiatrist asked me to examine her and see if the antidepressant medicine he had her taking was harming her.

Marie was educated, sophisticated, and wealthy. She was also lethargic, bored, and uninterested in life. I completed an extensive family and personal medical history, carefully examined her, and performed various tests. She was in fine physical condition. Her diet was fairly good: plenty of complex carbohydrates, vitamins, and minerals, not too much fat, sugar, salt, or junk foods. I recommended some changes in her diet and suggested she take a walk every morning and evening. She listlessly agreed. I called her psychiatrist to report my findings.

"Is her medication helping her depression?" I asked.

"Oh, it's holding her steady. At least she's not sinking further down," he answered.

"Why not try DLPA?" I said. "It can't hurt." He was familiar with DLPA and agreed to put her on 375 milligrams of DLPA twice a day. Three weeks later he called me. "She's a new woman. It's amazing!"

Marie was now energetic, lively, and arguing with him over his bill (something she never showed an interest in before). Where before she was laconic she now talked his ear off.

"I'm going to take her off the imipramine," he told me.

"I'm always a little uneasy about it, and if she doesn't need it there's no sense taking it."

Well, Marie is now free of depression for the first time in 30 years. She's interested in life, and in herself.

## HER HANDS DON'T SHAKE ANYMORE

A pretty young girl from Phoenix was brought to me by her mother. Toni, though petite and angelic looking, was also violent and angry. She fought with her siblings, parents, classmates, and teachers. Angry at everyone, she'd throw things at the wall—and at people. Although she had been to several psychiatrists and been on many medications, nothing seemed to help. Her mother hoped a nutritionally oriented physician like myself might help. I examined Toni and found her to be in excellent physical condition, except that her hands shook (tremor). It was a side effect of her medication. I spoke with Toni and her mother in my office.

"Except for the tremor there is nothing physically wrong with you. To make sure you stay healthy I'd like you to stop eating all that pizza, coke, and hamburgers, and get on a diet rich in complex carbohydrates, vitamins and minerals. I'd also like you to take DLPA, one tablet with breakfast. And come back in two weeks." Toni grunted.

Two weeks later she was back in my office. What a change! Before she was sullen and uncooperative—now she was quietly friendly. She even shook my hand.

"Dr. Fox, I didn't really eat what you told me to but I took the DLPA every day. Is that why I'm smiling?"

To make a long story short, Toni's psychiatrist and I agreed to slowly reduce her medication and increase her DLPA to two tablets a day. Within two months she was completely off her medication. I was very pleased to see that her hands stopped shaking. She became a shy, friendly youngster, and made friends in school.

## SELF-MEDICATION IS DANGEROUS

Toni and Marie are just two of the many people who have been helped by DLPA. But I do not want you to throw away your medicines or ignore your physician's advice. Discuss all changes in medication and/or therapy with your physician. I can recommend DLPA to patients I have carefully examined; but I never tell them to stop taking their other medications without first checking with their other doctors.

## HOW DOES DLPA WORK?

For more than 10 years medical researchers have been studying the biochemical effects of DL and D-phenylalanine. The research has provided some exciting insights into depression. Some of the promising explanations for DLPA's antidepressant effects include:

1. Protecting the endorphins
2. Raising phenylethylamine (PEA) levels in the brain
3. Increasing the manufacture of norepinephrine (NE) in the brain

## HYPOTHETICAL CONVERGENCE OF FACTORS CONTRIBUTING TO DLPA'S ANTIDEPRESSANT EFFECTS

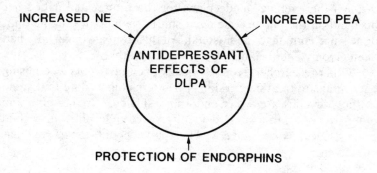

INCREASED NE

INCREASED PEA

ANTIDEPRESSANT EFFECTS OF DLPA

PROTECTION OF ENDORPHINS

Let's look at these theories.

## PROTECTING ENDORPHINS

We've known for many years that drugs derived from opium, such as morphine and heroin, induce feelings of euphoria. The endorphins are:

1. functionally very similar to morphine; and
2. are made in parts of the brain involved with emotions.

So it seems likely that endorphins might play a role in regulating mood.

Here is a dramatic example of the endorphin's ability to raise a person's mood. A team of researchers headed by Dr. Robert Gerner[8] in the Department of Psychiatry at the University of California, Los Angeles School of Medicine gave 10 milligrams of beta-endorphin to 10 severely depressed patients. In only 2 to 4 hours patients were feeling significant antidepressant effects.

Dr. Gerner told the story of one middle-aged woman who had spent most of her time sitting on the hospital ward or lying in bed. She rarely spoke with or played games with other patients. When she first received endorphins she said she did not think "anything would help."

A few hours later, without being asked, she told one of the researchers she must have been given "the real thing." She talked and played games with the other patients and hospital staff through the evening, made plans for the future, and called her husband on the phone. She even smiled, something she had not done since coming to the hospital. All this from a woman who had been gloomy and melancholy for three months!

Other researchers[9] report equally exciting results when using endorphins to treat depression. It's interesting to note that some of the tricyclics are weak endorphin shields.[10] Imipramine and other tricyclics, to a small degree, protect endorphins in certain brain tissues, as does DLPA. This may account in part for their effectiveness.

## RAISING PEA

DL-phenylalanine might also relieve depression by raising phenylethylamine (PEA) levels. Phenylethylamine is a neurotransmitter closely related to norepinephrine (NE). As you will learn in chapter 12, PEA is derived from DLPA.

Brain scientists have found a strong link between PEA and depression. Study after study has shown that depressed patients have much lower levels of PEA in body fluids than nondepressed patients. Researchers also found that most antidepression therapies, including the drugs, raise PEA levels. This suggests that the therapies might owe part of their effectiveness to their ability to raise endorphin levels.[11]

Well, if low levels of PEA are associated with depression, what is the safest and most effective way to raise PEA? DL-phenylalanine might be the answer. A series of studies[12] has reported a striking correlation between depression, PEA levels, and PA (either DPA or DLPA). It seems that giving DLPA or DPA to depressed patients raises their PEA levels *and* relieves their depression.

## INCREASING NE

A third possibility is that DLPA relieves depression by increasing the amount of the brain stimulant NE manufactured in the brain.

There are drugs to protect NE levels, of course, but they have side effects. Is there a safer way to get the brain to produce more NE?

The brain can use two common amino acids, L-phenylalanine and L-tyrosine to make NE. Some researchers felt that if you "loaded up" with these two amino acids by eating large amounts, the brain would make more NE. It is an interesting idea, but there is no way to guarantee the "loaded" amino acids will get to the right parts of the brain and be transformed into NE. They are more likely to be "grabbed up" for other duties in the body, such as protein synthesis. There are no published studies showing L-phenylalanine "loading" helps depression. Several recent studies suggest L-tyrosine helps, but these studies involved only a few patients, while other studies showed negative results.

But DLPA may succeed where the other two failed because DLPA, or rather, the D- component, is more likely to get into the right parts of the brain and eventually be converted into NE than L-phenylalanine and L-tyrosine are. That's because DPA is less likely to be "grabbed up" for other duties, and has a relatively easier time crossing into the brain.

## "THE VERY ECSTASY OF LOVE"?

Is there a "love pill" in our future? Some prominent scientists feel that PEA is the chief suspect in the search for the biochemical source of the falling-in-love euphoria.

Sages throughout the ages have sought to answer Cole Porter's question; "What is this thing called love?" Is that invigorating, exhilarating, enlivening, and elating feeling caused by chemical changes in the brain? Can we "create" love by mixing the right chemicals together in the laboratory?

There is a lot of PEA in chocolate, but don't buy 900 pounds of chocolate candy for the reluctant object of your desires. Dr. Donald Klein and Dr. Michael Liebowitz[13] of the New York State Psychiatric Institute, specialists in the neurochemistry of emotions who put forth the "PEA hypothesis of the neurochemistry of love," are not claiming that PEA is a love potion. What they do say is that sharp rises in PEA activity in the brain cause the feelings of "falling in love."

But now the key question is: What causes the PEA to become more active? And, what other chemicals are active in your brain whilst you and your loved one sip champagne from each other's slippers?

We know that DLPA can be converted in the brain into PEA, and PEA is associated with those euphoric feelings of newfound love. Will future would-be Romeos be slipping DLPA into their loved one's drink?

# 5

# DR. FOX'S DLPA ANTIDEPRESSION PLAN

Karen first came to see me when she was 35 years old, so depressed she seriously considered suicide. She told a story I've heard many times before. She "went through" medical school with her husband; that is, he attended class, studied every night, and worked on the weekends. She worked during the day and sat home alone at night. Occasionally they found time to spend together, but he was invariably tired from work and school. Far from home and very shy, Karen had no close friends with whom to share a movie or a talk. So far Karen's depression seemed to be reactive; she was depressed because she was lonely. But as she went on to explain:

"I kept thinking, just a few more years, he'll graduate and we can go home. We'll be back home with our families and friends. Dave (her husband) finally finished and we went home to set up his practice. We were back with our families, friends, Dave and I spent a lot of time together, we had children, we even bought the house I wanted since I was 10. But I was still depressed. All those years I thought I was depressed because I was lonely. Then I wasn't lonely anymore—but I was still depressed! I don't know what it is, Dr. Fox. I have everything I dreamed of—more. But nothing matters. Everything is boring. Everything."

I put Karen on my DLPA Antidepression Plan. I asked her to change to the Antistress Diet, strengthen her Mental Blueprints, and take DLPA. I emphasized the Mental Blueprints, and strongly encouraged her to PA Walk every day. A very intelligent and well-educated woman, Karen asked many very sophisticated questions about DLPA and the Antidepression Plan. Two weeks later she came back to my office for a follow-up examination. She told me she was following the Antidepression Plan and felt good. I did not hear from her for a while, until her husband called me.

"She's been in bed all week, she won't get up. She hasn't been following your instructions. The bottle of DLPA you gave her was never opened and she's eating the same diet she always did."

The next day I had a long discussion with Karen, her husband, and her children. We carefully reviewed my DLPA Antidepression Plan and worked out strategies to help Karen stick with it. It has been an uphill battle all the way, but with her husband and children supporting her, Karen eventually managed to follow my guidelines. Now, after six months of adherence to the Antidepression Plan, Karen says:

"I'm so happy Dave and the kids loved me enough to make me stay on your program, Dr. Fox. For the first time in years I feel like I want to keep on living forever."

## FIGHTING BACK FOUR WAYS

Like my DLPA Antipain Plan, Dr. Fox's DLPA Antidepression Plan attacks the enemy from all directions, with:

DIET: The Antistress Diet features complex carbohydrates; plus aloe, vitamins, and minerals to build the best of health.

MENTAL BLUEPRINTS: Visualization and affirmations to design positive Mental Blueprints strong enough to support depression-free health and happiness.

EXERCISE: PA Walking or other PA aerobic exercise for building body and Mental Blueprints simultaneously.

DLPA: Protection for your endorphins.

In chapter 3 I covered the general principles of Dr. Fox's DLPA Program. The basic program for treating depression is the same. In this section I will focus on aspects particularly important for dealing with depression.

## HOLIDAY HEART

It's been hectic at work and you're looking forward to the three-day weekend. Friday night you and your spouse have dinner with another couple; you drink cocktails and wine. Saturday night it's dinner and a show; more cocktails and wine. On Sunday the home team is on television; beer. Monday it's a family picnic and baseball game; more beer.

In four days you have had more to drink than you normally have in a month. What's the effect of all that alcohol? Had you been watching a monitor attached to your heart that weekend, you might have seen your heart palpating and beating with rapid, irregular rhythms. (Irregular rhythms can be fatal.) It's what we call Holiday Heart.

> I saw one patient, a 49-year-old man, when he was brought to the emergency room clutching his chest. "Doctor," he gasped. "It was beating like crazy. It wouldn't stop!" Normally a moderate drinker, this man had spent the weekend drinking with "the boys." By the second day he could literally feel his heart pounding away.

There is an enzyme in your liver called alcohol dehydrogenase. Its job is to "defuse" alcohol in your body. But when you drink large amounts, you overwhelm the liver's ability to produce that enzyme. It cannot keep up. One of alcohol's breakdown products is acetaldehyde. Acetaldehyde stimulates your adrenal medulla (part of your adrenal glands) and liberates catecholamines (chemical substances, such as adrenalin). This creates dangerous stress—especially for your heart.

## AFTER-HOLIDAY BLUES

The drinking that causes "Holiday Heart" may also lead to After-Holiday blues. Alcohol is a depressant: That's the last thing a depressed person needs. I tell my depressed patients that it is best not to drink any alcohol at all. I limit those who feel they *must* have some to one drink a day.

One day, several years ago, I instructed a patient to limit himself to one drink a day. The next day his angry wife called me demanding to know why I told her husband to drink a full quart of vodka a day! Apparently the gentleman misunderstood my instructions. One alcoholic drink a day means *no more than*:

1½ ounces of hard liquor, straight or mixed, *or*
4 ounces of wine, *or*
12 ounces of beer

But it is best to do without. Alcohol is a stressor, a depressant, and is full of empty calories.

## SUGAR DRAGON

The middle-aged man sitting in my office was listless and unresponsive. He stared at his feet, answering my questions with grunts. When I finally got him to talk he limited his discourse to two sentences: "Life's boring. It's always boring."

Was he depressed? You bet! With the man's permission I performed an experiment. I had him eat a piece of pie and drink some coke. Forty-five minutes later I thought I was talking to a different person. He was supercharged with energy and excitement: "Who decorated your office? It's nice. A little dark maybe, but nice. One of my cousins is a decorator. I'll have him come and see if he can lighten up your place a bit. No charge. Not for a friend. You know, I've only known you for a little while but it seems like we've been friends for years. . . ." He jabbered without a rest for 30 minutes, then slowed down and sank back into a sullen, almost catatonic silence.

This man was a victim of the Sugar Dragon. He ate the Standard American Diet (SAD) which is full of highly refined carbohydrates. These highly refined carbohydrates are nothing more than sugar. He ate pizza, pasta, white bread, soda, candy, cake, and ice cream. Eating those sugary foods brought the Sugar Dragon out bellowing and blowing fire. That's when he was excited and full of fiery energy. But then the Sugar Dragon ran out of fire and slunk back into its dark cave. Suddenly the man had no energy. He plopped down into a chair and sat there like a rag doll. His wife told me he was like that all day, alternating between short periods of intense energy, and very long periods of apathetic lethargy.

Sugar worsens depression by picking you up, then throwing you down—hard. I tell my patients to stop eating sugar and sugary foods. Stay away from refined carbohydrates like white flour products, processed foods, cakes, candy, soda, ice cream, and pie. Stick with the complex carbohydrates in fresh vegetables and whole grains. (In chapter 9 I will discuss the Sugar Dragon in greater detail.)

## A PHONY LIFT

Then there is caffeine. Depressed people are usually tired, so a cup of coffee should pick them up, right? Wrong. Just like sugar, caffeine lifts you up, then drops you down. Caffeine stimulates the adrenal glands, setting in motion a sugarlike reaction. You get the Sugar Dragon, even though you did not eat sugar.

You drink caffeine for the lift, but soon you are more tired than before. So you have some more, but soon you are tired again. For many of my patients it is an endless cycle of caffeine, lift, and crash. Trying to beat the caffeine crashes with more caffeine does not work.

One of the "caffeine crash" patients I treated was a 28-year-old wife and mother of two small children. Her husband told me that since the second child was born his wife had absolutely no energy. The kids were not being taken care of properly, he told me, and the house was always a mess. He thought that her constant fatigue was related to her second pregnancy.

As soon as I found out how much coffee she drank I suspected her second pregnancy was not responsible for her fatigue—it was the caffeine. This woman drank an average of 20 cups of coffee a day!

"As soon as I wake up I have a cup of coffee, it helps me get going." Getting her to cut back to two cups of coffee a day wasn't easy—but it was worth it. She has a lot more energy now that she's not drinking all that coffee.

Caffeine will fool you, trap you into drinking more and more in a fruitless attempt to beat fatigue. Caffeine worsens depression by making already tired people even more tired.

On top of that, caffeine can cause dangerous irregular heart rhythms. I have seen this many times in my patients. Once I monitored the effects of caffeine on my own heart. I drank two cups of coffee and had my electrocardiogram (a measure of the heart) taken every half hour for 4 hours. The number of irregular heart beats caused by just two cups of coffee was enough to convince me to stay away from caffeine.

Caffeine robs you of energy and harms your heart. Stay away from coffee, tea, soft drinks, cocoa, chocolate, and other foods containing caffeine. Beware of hidden caffeine: It shows up in places you may not expect it; for example, Excedrin, Midol, Vanquish, and Anacin. (Ask your physician or pharmacist before you take prescription or nonprescription drugs if they have caffeine. If they do, ask for an alternative medicine.)

Fill your plate, and your body, with fresh vegetables, fruits, whole grain, seeds, and small amounts of low-fat fish, poultry, and dairy products. Give yourself the complex carbohydrates, fiber, vitamins, and minerals you need to build your towers of stress-free health.

## ALOE VERA JUICE

Add to your general health with aloe vera juice, that excellent general tonic and promoter of good health. Aloe contains a good supply of many necessary nutrients. Just as for the Antipain Plan, I have my patients on the Antidepression Plan start with 2 ounces of aloe vera juice every day with breakfast. I like to drink it mixed with apple juice. Patients slowly add more aloe vera until they reach bowel tolerance (loose stools). I start my patients on this schedule:

**Day 1:**  2 ounces with breakfast
**Day 4:**  Add 2 ounces with lunch
**Day 7:**  Add 2 ounces with dinner
They are now taking 2 ounces three times a day
They continue on with this dosage until;
**Day 15:** Add 2 ounces to the breakfast dose
**Day 18:** Add 2 ounces to the lunch dose
**Day 21:** Add 2 ounces to the dinner dose
They are now taking 4 ounces three times a day

If they can take more, great.

## VITAMIN C FOR DEPRESSION

Before describing the supplementation program I put my patients on, I'd like to tell you about one depressed man who was helped by vitamin C.

Mr. N. R., a 65-year-old man, had a coronary bypass surgery 6 months before I saw him. His chest pain, both before and after the operation, was so severe he was taking narcotic painkillers.

Things went from bad to worse after the operation. He developed severe depression and anorexia (loss of appetite.) He vomited often. His weight fell from 145 pounds to 104 pounds in a few months. This man's son, an actor and a friend of mine, asked me to examine his father.

It was obvious that the man was malnourished, but the question was why? Was the depression responsible for his anorexia? As I was examining him I thought about the groundbreaking study on depression and vitamin C performed by Drs. Kinsman and Hood. They found that depression occurred in every single patient whose vitamin C level was reduced by one-third. This man was not eating much at all, so he was probably low in vitamin C. I drew some of his blood for vitamin C and other tests. On that day, and the next day, I gave him vitamin C intravenously. I asked him to take vitamin C supplements and come back in a week to discuss my findings and recommendations.

A few days later his son called me to report that his father was no longer depressed and was eating with gusto. The problem seemed to have cleared up.

By the way, the lab reports came back the next day. They showed that the man did indeed have low blood levels of vitamin C before I gave him the vitamin C intravenously. (His level was 0.05 mg%. The average range is 0.2 to 2.0 mg%. I like to see it between 1.5 and 2.0 mg%.)

A year has passed. The man has recovered from his depression, he's eating well, has regained his weight, and his vitamin C levels are high.

## ANTIDEPRESSION SUPPLEMENTS

Every individual is unique. Nutrient requirements vary from one person to the next, and I cannot prescribe vitamins and minerals without first examining a person. This is the nutrient regimen I have most of my depression patients start with:

**VITAMIN A**—I tell my patients to eat two or three carrots a day, and lots of green vegetables, orange vegetables, and orange fruit during the week. These foods contain beta-carotene, which is converted to vitamin A in your body.

**B COMPLEX**—A B-complex vitamin containing 50 mg of the major B vitamins and 400 mcgm of folic acid. Take one tablet or capsule twice a day.

In addition to the B complex, I suggest that my depressed patients take these B vitamins:

**NIACINAMIDE**—500 mg three times a day. Niacinamide is a form of vitamin $B_3$.

**NIACIN**—Niacin is also a form of vitamin $B_3$. I have my depressed patients take niacin according to this schedule:
    **Week 1:** 50 mg, three times a day, with meals
    **Week 2:** 100 mg, three times a day, with meals
    **Week 3:** 150 mg, three times a day, with meals
    **Week 4:** 200 mg, three times a day, with meals

They are then to stay at the higher dosage. If at any time an uncomfortable flushing of the face or body develops, I instruct them to drop down to the next lower dosage.

**PANTOTHENIC ACID**—500 mg of pantothenic acid (or calcium pantothenate) three times a day. Pantothenic acid is also known as Vitamin $B_5$.

**PYRIDOXINE**—50 mg three times a day. Pyridoxine is also known as vitamin $B_6$.

**VITAMIN C**—I have my patients taking two types of this vitamin. First is buffered vitamin C powder (ph 6.3). They take 1 teaspoon in water (or juice) with breakfast, which provides:

| | |
|---|---|
| Vitamin C | 2,350 mg |
| Calcium | 450 mg |
| Magnesium | 250 mg |
| Potassium | 99 mg |

In addition to the buffered form, I have them take 2,000 mg of vitamin C in tablet form three times a day. Preferably, these should be taken at 8-hour intervals, or as close to this as is possible.

Between the powdered and tablet forms, my patients take 4,350 mg vitamin C in the morning, 2,000 mg in the afternoon, and 2,000 mg at night.

**VITAMIN E**—400 mg of D-alpha tocopheral (vitamin E) twice a day.

**MINERALS**—I have my patients begin with a multiple mineral that contains 1/4 of the recommended daily allowance (RDAs) for all the minerals, and take four tablets a day—two tablets twice daily.

In addition to the multiminerals, I suggest these to my patients:

**CALCIUM CARBONATE**—1,000 mg calcium carbonate with 400 mg vitamin D a day, at bedtime.

**MAGNESIUM**—400 mg, at bedtime.

**MANGANESE**—15 mg, three times a day. Manganese theoretically improves a person's memory. Some positive studies support this theory.

**ZINC**—220 mg of zinc sulfate twice a day. Zinc helps the memory and depression.

**TRYPTOPHAN**—500 mg capsules, twice a day. Once at 8 A.M. and once at 8 P.M. Tryptophan is an essential amino acid which your body needs to manufacture serotonin, a neurotransmitter which helps regulate mood. Low serotonin levels can bring on depression and help cause insomnia.

This is the basic antidepression supplementation plan, which I vary according to individual needs. When the DLPA Antidepression Plan has helped my patients to feel really good, I have them reduce their supplements, step by step, back down to the basic supplementation plan outlined in chapter 3.

## REWRITE DEPRESSED MENTAL BLUEPRINTS

Now let's look at Mental Blueprints and depression. Depressed people have "unhappy" and "miserable" and "terrible" scrawled all over their Mental Blueprints. These negative Blueprints are shaky, not a strong foundation for your towers of good health. Strengthen your foundation by rewriting your Mental Blueprints. I tell my patients to go into a quiet room where they will not be disturbed, to practice "saying their depression away."

You cannot be happy unless you believe you are happy. That is the basic premise. And you cannot believe you are happy unless your Mental Blueprints are filled with happiness.

Affirmations are the best way to "write" happiness all over your Mental Blueprints. Here is an antidepression affirmation I have my patients say:

I am happy!
I give myself permission to enjoy myself.
I give myself permission to enjoy life.
Being alive is being happy.
I am alive *and I am happy*!

I instruct them to repeat it over and over again, silently to themselves, then out loud. Here is another affirmation I give them:

Everywhere I look I see happiness:
In a child's laugh
A lover's smile
A flower
A park
A sunset
A friend
and in me.
There is happiness everywhere,
especially in me.
I cannot help but be happy.

While they're saying their affirmations I have my patients visualize their depression away. I tell them to picture a piece of paper in their mind's eye. That paper is their Mental Blueprint. The word *unhappy* is written all over the Mental Blueprint, covering it so completely there is no room to write anything else. I tell them to see their hand, holding an eraser, deliberately and firmly erasing all the *unhappy's,* one by one, until their Mental Blueprint is clean. Next, I have them imagine their hand is holding a pen and writing in big, bold strokes on the Mental Blueprint:

I am happy!
I give myself permission to enjoy myself.
I give myself permission to enjoy life.
Being alive is being happy.
I am alive *and I am happy!*

I ask my depressed patients to picture themselves doing the things that make them happy. If going to the park makes you happy, picture yourself in the park. It's a sunny spring day, the grass is cool and green, trees are colored by leaves, children are playing. You are with the people you love. Imagine that one of your friends is telling a joke. Picture youself laughing at the joke. Now imagine that you are telling a joke. All your friends laugh along with you as you give the punch line. See it in your mind's eye; you and your friends laughing together. Picture yourself enjoying life.

Say it and see it with affirmations and visualizations. Pretty soon you'll feel it.

## MOVING FOR A "LIFT"

Exercise is a great mood lifter. Your body was made to move and moving is fun. PA Walking, PA Jogging, PA Aerobic Dancing, and the other PA exercises strengthen your mind and body at the same time. Here is another affirmation you can repeat to yourself while PA exercising:

I enjoy living!
I enjoy being!
I enjoy exercising!
I enjoy being myself!

Repeat this and other affirmations over and over in your mind as you PA exercise. Remember, you're PA exercising for fun and health, you're not trying to break the Olympic record—just have fun.

## DLPA FOR DEPRESSION

Now I'll complete Dr. Fox's Antidepression Plan by adding the DLPA. This is the basic schedule I start my patients on:

**375 Milligrams of DLPA Twice a Day**

375 milligrams with breakfast
375 milligrams with lunch

I instruct my patients to have regular meals: breakfast at 8 A.M., lunch at noon. DLPA should be taken with the meal, or within an hour after completing the meal. I prefer it to be taken 5 minutes after the meal. On the third day I generally have patients increase the dosage to:

### 375 Milligrams of DLPA Three Times a Day

375 milligrams with breakfast
375 milligrams with lunch
375 milligrams with dinner

Again, I tell my patients to have regular meals: breakfast at 8 A.M., lunch at noon, and dinner between 5 and 6 P.M. DLPA should be taken with the meal, or within an hour after completing the meal. I prefer it to be taken five minutes after finishing the meal. *It is very important that dinner be finished by 6 P.M. and DLPA be taken shortly after.* If my patients have trouble sleeping at night because DLPA gives them a feeling of excitement or energy, I have them cut the dinner dose in half. This is the basic plan, which I vary to meet the needs of individual patients. I carefully monitor their progress, adjusting the dosage up or down as needed.

NOTE: *You do not have to stop taking any medications prescribed by your doctor to benefit from DLPA.*

*I tell My Patients to Stay with DLPA—Give It a Chance To Work.*

My observation has been that it takes anywhere from five days to three weeks for DLPA to reduce the symptoms of depression. It may take as long as four to six weeks, so I encourage my patients not to get discouraged. DLPA is not fast acting. It takes *at least* five days to have effect. Give it a chance to work! When they have felt really good for a full week, I have my patients stop taking DLPA and wait for the symptoms to recur. They go on an alternating schedule, taking DLPA until they feel good for a full week, then not taking it until the symptoms reappear, and so on. Many of my patients only use DLPA one out of every three or four weeks. Patients are encouraged to adjust their dosage in consultation with their physician.

CAUTION: *I recommend against using DLPA during pregnancy or lactation. Pregnant or lactating women should not expose the fetus or newborn to anything except their normal diet. It's best to be safe. Neither should any person suffering from the genetic disease phenyeketonuria (PKU) take DLPA—they cannot metabolize phenylalanine normally. This also applies to those on a phenylalanine-restricted diet. Neither do I recommend the use of DLPA for children under the age of 14. I arbitrarily chose this age because as an internist and cardiologist I do not usually treat children. However, physicians experienced in treating children may wish to examine the DLPA literature. They may find an appropriate use for DLPA, such as in juvenile rheumatoid arthritis.*

## ITS A PACKAGE PLAN

All parts of Dr. Fox's DLPA Antidepression Plan are important. The Antistress Diet, Mental Blueprints, PA Walking, and DLPA all have a role to play. Give them a chance to work together and contribute to your good health.

## DO NOT SELF-MEDICATE

Do not throw away the medicine(s) your doctor has prescribed for you. Do not alter the dosage or stop taking the medicine(s). Discuss DLPA and Dr. Fox's DLPA Program with your physician. A trained professional, your physician will be able to guide you through the intricacies of the human body and mind. The nice thing about DLPA is that it does not interfere with other medication. You and your doctor can try DLPA without stopping your other medications. My experience with my patients has been that with DLPA I can carefully reduce my patient's other medicines, and often eliminate them entirely.

## "TALKY PILL"

"DLPA? I call it my talky pill because it made me talk again. Did you know I had nothing, not a thing to say for five years? I was so depressed I didn't talk to anyone. Not my husband, not my kids, not my friends. I didn't even go out of the house. *Doing* anything was too depressing. I used to stare at the ceiling a lot. I know how many tiles there are on every ceiling in my house." This delightful and energetic 62-year-old woman, named Gert, actually told me how many tiles there were on every ceiling in her house.

For years her husband dragged her to different doctors and psychologists, making her take the various antidepressant drugs that were prescribed. She came to me because she had nausea and was vomiting. These were side effects of her medication. Her psychiatrist and I agreed to give her DLPA while she was still on her drugs. In two weeks we could see a clear improvement in her mood. She smiled occasionally, spoke without being prompted, and took an interest in her appearance. Her doctor and I increased her DLPA dosage, took her off the drugs and put her on my DLPA Antidepression Plan. Within two months she was her old vivacious self again, going to parties, visiting her children (who lived in another state), and making plans for the future.

# 6

# ARTHRITIS: INFLAMING CRIPPLER

## "MOVEAPHOBIC"

"Dr. Fox, is there a word for someone who is afraid to move? 'Moveaphobic' maybe? Because I'm a 'moveaphobic.' I'll move my head, neck, hands, fingers, and legs, but not my shoulders, my back, or my waist. I can't. It hurts too much!

"It's a good thing I'm a writer and work at home or I couldn't support myself. When I get out of bed in the morning I go right to my desk and sit down and stay sitting for the whole day. I've got wheels on my chair—it's not a wheelchair but it has little wheels, you know, on the legs. I've got my house set up with everything I need near my desk; the fridge, all my books, telephone, TV, even a little urine bottle so I don't have to get up to go to the bathroom all the time. This arthritis has ruined my life. I used to play volleyball and racquetball, go dancing once in a while. Now I sit on my rear at my desk all day and get fat. What kind of life is that? This has been going on for three years, Dr. Fox. Have you got some new wonder drug for me?"

## THE COSTS?

According to the Arthritis Foundation:[1]

- More than 36 million American suffer from arthritis.
- 1 of every 7 Americans has arthritis.
- Arthritis hits 1 in every 3 families.

We cannot put a dollar sign on the pain and suffering, but we can total up the bill for arthritis care. Every year we spend:

- $5,428,000,000 on medical care for arthritis
- $798,000,000 on arthritis drugs

The total direct costs of medical care for arthritis come to $6,226,000,000 each and every year!

The indirect costs are just as staggering:

- $6,046,000,000 in lost wages every year.
- $661,000,000 in lost homemaker services

The total indirect costs of arthritis add up to $7,043,000,000 a year, and the grand total of all the direct and indirect costs of arthritis to this country comes to $13,269,000,000 each and every year!

That is an incredible sum of money. I can't even picture that much money. But I have seen many patients who would gladly pay twice that amount to get rid of their arthritis pain!

## "ARTH" + "ITIS"

The word *arthritis* means "inflamed joint": Arth = joint, and itis = inflammation. But we use the word *arthritis* as a general term that includes over 100 different illnesses. There is osteoarthritis, rheumatoid arthritis, gouty arthritis, juvenile rheumatoid arthritis, bursitis, infectious arthritis, systemic lupus erythematosus, ankylosing spondylitis, psoratic arthritis, arthritis associated with venereal disease, and many other forms of this sometimes very painful and crippling disease.

## IS THERE A CURE?

At the present time there is no cure for arthritis; especially when the bone or cartilage has degenerated, there is not a whole lot we can do. Surgery or joint replacement is helpful in some cases, but for many millions of sufferers conventional medicine offers little relief.

## RELIEVING PAIN *AND* INFLAMMATION

No, we cannot cure arthritis, but we can help with the pain and inflammation. I must stress that relieving pain and inflammation *is not a cure* for arthritis. But if we can give arthritis victims back the use of their fingers, hands, shoulders, legs, and back; if we can unlock their frozen joints; if we can make it possible for them to live without constant pain; if we can do this we would restore some sense of normality to their lives.

Patient after patient has told me they could learn to live with their arthritis if only it didn't hurt so much, if only their hands were not so swollen, if only they could carry on their daily lives. As Alex C., a retired clerk, said:

> "Since I retired two years ago, what I like to do is make things for my grandchildren and friends. I have a little wood shop in my garage—nothing fancy—and I make little toys for my grandchildren. I make them little trucks, dolls. I make things for my friends too. It's not a big deal, but it's what I do." Six months ago his hands became swollen with rheumatoid arthritis.
>
> "I can't hold the tools anymore. My youngest granddaughter, Melanie, her birthday is next month. How can I make her a present if I can't hold the tools?"

Alex's woodwork, making gifts for his grandchildren, was his life. Arthritic inflammation made woodworking impossible.

Lillian O., a 62-year-old widow, was concerned with the pain of arthritis in her fingers.

"I volunteer at the Children's Hospital," she told me. "I used to be a piano teacher. And I'd play for the children in the hospital. Two years ago my back started hurting with arthritis—the doctor told me the name but I can't remember. I take three different pills; a blue one, a red one, and a white one. But my back still always hurts. It hurts so much I can't play for the children anymore."

## DRUGS AND SIDE EFFECTS

Many drugs are designed to reduce pain and inflammation. Here are just a few of them: aspirin, Tylenol, Darvon, Empirin with codeine, Clinoril, Indocin, Motrin, Tolectin, Nalfon, Meclomen, and Trilisate. There are very strong narcotic pain killers such as Demerol and Percodan. Immunosuppressant drugs such as Cytoxan and Leukeran are occasionally used in severe cases of rheumatoid arthritis and other forms of arthritis. These drugs help many people by relieving pain and inflammation. But with arthritis drugs, as with all drugs, you run the risk of side effects— sometimes very serious ones.

Cortisone and cortisonelike drugs were first used in the 1950's for rheumatoid arthritis. These drugs, helpful for a while, become very dangerous over longer periods of time. They suppress the immune system, leaving the patient open to possibly serious infections and other problems. The immunosuppressants may cause liver damage, suppression of white blood cells, and possibly even cancer. This is what Naprosyn and Tolectin, two of the more popular arthritic drugs, may do:

NAPROSYN—a nonsteroidal (noncortisone) antiinflammatory drug

About 20 percent of the patients I have seen who were taking Naprosyn suffered from side effects. The most frequent problem is bleeding into the stomach. Other problems include nausea, dyspepsia, abdominal pain, bloody bowel movements, and diarrhea.

     **TOLECTIN**—This medication causes a wide variety of problems ranging from ulcers to high blood pressure. I've treated patients for Tolectin-induced headaches, chest pain, bloating, depression, vomiting, intestinal distress, bleeding stomachs, and high blood pressure.

The narcotics, such as Empirin with codeine, Percodan, and Darvon, kill pain but can be addicting. Injections of gold salts are used for some cases of severe arthritis. Gold salts can damage the kidneys and suppress the body's ability to make blood. In an earlier chapter I discussed the lethal side effects of Oroflex, a drug no longer on the market.

## NO PAIN—BUT LOTS OF BLOOD

     I'll never forget the pleasant, placid, but very tired 70-year-old man who came to see me. "I'm so tired," he said, over and over. He was taking Tolectin for his arthritis. It really helped reduce his pain. But when I checked his stool I found it contained blood. He was painlessly bleeding from his stomach. Losing all that blood lowered his red blood cell count and made him severely anemic and constantly tired. The bleeding stopped when I put him in the hospital and took him off his arthritis medication. I put him on DLPA for his arthritis and he's doing fine.

## STRANGLING YOUR OWN IMMUNE SYSTEM

     Back in 1975 a female patient of mine called to say she had had a sore throat for two weeks. I told her to come to my office so I could take a look at it.

     Her throat was not red and she had no fever. She told me she had just come back from a two-month trip to New York City. Her arthritis flared up while she was there, so a local doctor gave her Butazolidin (phenylbutazone). Knowing about the possible adverse reactions to this drug, I checked her blood. The blood count confirmed my suspicions: Her bone marrow and white blood cells were severely depressed, seriously compromising her immune system, and increasing her risk of "catching" all kinds of diseases. Butazolidin helps with arthritis, but has too many side effects! I took her off this medication and kept her in "reverse" isolation in the hospital. People coming into her room had to wear surgical masks over their faces and surgical gowns over their clothes so she wouldn't "catch" a disease. Seven anxious days passed before her white blood count rose enough to be considered safe. She recovered and is now doing fine.

## THE SAFE AND EFFECTIVE ALTERNATIVE IS DLPA

Three of the 10 participants in the original DPA/pain study were treated for arthritis pain. D-phenylalanine effectively relieved their pain, and loosened up the joint stiffness in one. This was a pain study, not an arthritis study, but it suggested that DL-phenylalanine might be useful in treating arthritis.

Two of the major problems arthritis patients have to deal with are pain and inflammation. D-phenylalanine had been shown to relieve many types of chronic pain, as well as arthritis pain specifically. Would it also reduce inflammation?

A team of researchers created an arthritislike state of painful inflammation in laboratory animals by injecting them with carageenin. (Carageenin is a chemical which causes extremely severe inflammatory reactions when injected under the skin.) DLPA significantly reduced the inflammation in about 78% of the animals![2] And in a later study the researchers stated that DPA is a very effective anti-inflammatory agent.[3] And in 1983 Dr. Balagot of the Chicago Medical School published the results of his study[4] in which DPA proved to be a particularly effective treatment for arthritis symptoms, especially for "those suffering from osteoarthritic disease." (30 of the 43 participants in this study had osteoarthritis).

## DLPA IS SAFE

DLPA is an effective alternative to the arthritis drugs. How about safety? Here is a comparison of the toxicity of DLPA and commonly used arthritis drugs.

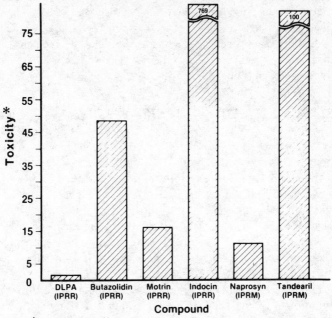

**ACUTE TOXICITY OF DL-PHENYLALANINE
COMPARED WITH COMMONLY USED
ARTHRITIS DRUGS**

\* 1/LD 50 (x10⁻⁴)

## DLPA IS LONG LASTING

Safe and effective, DLPA is also long lasting. Compare how long DLPA works to relieve arthritis to some commonly used arthritis drugs:

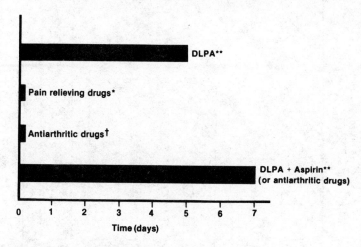

**AVERAGE DURATION OF ACTION OF DLPA
COMPARED TO PAIN RELIEVING DRUGS AND
ANTIARTHRITIC DRUGS**

*Average of 5 commonly prescribed analgesic drugs
†Average of 5 commonly prescribed antiarthritic drugs
**Estimate based on published values and clinical experience.

## DLPA IS LESS EXPENSIVE IN THE LONG RUN

DLPA is less expensive than other common arthritis drugs, except aspirin. But remember, once you are on the on/off schedule, you're not taking DLPA every day. You might only take it one out of every three weeks. Aspirin and the other arthritis medications have to be taken one or more times a day.

The chart below shows the average retail cost for a 30-day supply. You will likely be taking DLPA for only a fraction of those days, so your average *daily* cost is much lower.

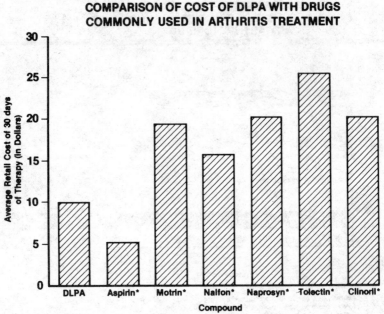

COMPARISON OF COST OF DLPA WITH DRUGS COMMONLY USED IN ARTHRITIS TREATMENT

*Values from The Family Physician's Compendium of Drug Therapy, 1981

## HOW DOES DLPA WORK AGAINST ARTHRITIS?

DLPA's combined pain-blocking and antiinflammatory actions are striking, and seem to involve the endorphin system at different parts of the body. You have already learned how DLPA blocks pain. How about the inflammation? Our present scientific evidence suggests that the enkephalins or "small endorphins" can reduce severe, experimentally induced arthritislike inflammation. Your body produces prostaglandins (hormones) which play a role in producing inflammation. Reporting in the journal *Prostaglandins*,[5] Drs. Ferreira and Nakamura found that the enkephalins could block the inflammatory effects of the prostaglandins. This and other studies have not fixed the exact mechanisms by which DLPA reduces the symptoms of arthritis, but they point the way for possible future research.

## "IT DIDN'T COME BACK"

Now that we have taken a brief look at the DLPA–endorphin–arthritis studies, let's look at a DLPA case history.

Beatrice is a 73-year-old woman who developed arthritis after having knee surgery 7 years ago. "Oh, my arthritis wasn't as bad as some people's, Dr. Fox. But it kept me from walking to the park. I love to go to the park and watch the children play. My daughter bought me a cane to walk with, but it was still hard to walk to the park. The doctor gave me lots of pills. All I got from them was an upset stomach and I was sleepy all day. They didn't help my arthritis much. This new pill you gave me (DLPA) is wonderful. I think my arthritis has improved 75 percent. I walk to the park every day without my cane now.

"Three weeks ago I ran out of DLPA. I was afraid of the arthritis coming back. Without the DLPA I *knew* it would come back. My daughter was out of town so I had no one to take me to the store for more. I was so frantic!

"You'll think I'm so silly, but I'll tell you what happened. The next morning when I woke up I was afraid to move. I didn't move a muscle because I didn't want my knee to hurt me again. It was so nice being able to move it. I didn't want it to hurt again. I stayed in bed 45 minutes without moving because I knew it would hurt. But I had to go to the bathroom. You know what? My knee didn't hurt! I moved it, stood up, walked, stomped my foot on the ground, but I couldn't make my knee hurt! I didn't hurt for eight days! Now I use DLPA for a week then don't use it for two weeks. It doesn't hurt during the two weeks."

Now let's look at the practical application; Dr. Fox's DLPA Antiarthritis Plan.

# 7

# DR. FOX'S DLPA ANTIARTHRITIS PLAN

"DLPA is my favorite subject. I tell everyone about it. All the time. I talk so much about it they think I'm crazy but I don't care. I want to tell everybody about it." This 54-year-old woman had suffered from what she described as "terrible" back and leg pain caused by arthritis in her lower back.

"I couldn't dance anymore, I couldn't walk, I could barely stand up. I spent years going from doctor to doctor. I took pills, pills, I don't remember how many different pills. If I listed the side effects they gave me it would be a whole book. I had four back surgeries. I even had electrodes put in my brain. Stimulating my brain was supposed to stop my back pain. It didn't work. There were complications, the wires came out of place. They had to take them out."

A person willing to put up with four surgeries and the placement of brain electrodes must be in great pain. I put her on Dr. Fox's DLPA Antiarthritis Plan, quickly building her up to six tablets of DL-phenylalanine a day. Because her pain was so severe I also had her taking aspirin to complement and strengthen the DLPA. By the end of the third week she experienced almost complete pain relief. She is now on an on/off schedule: one week on, two weeks off.

"I tell everyone I know about it. Even people I don't know I tell about it. All right, maybe I'm crazy. But I'll keep telling everyone."

## JOINT-CRUSHING FAT

Imagine that there is a 50-pound weight sitting right on top of your head. It's glued on, you can't take it off. Now walk around—it's hard, isn't it? Your knees keep buckling, it is hard to keep your back straight, your muscles ache.

We do not have 50-pound weights attached to our heads, of course. But many of us have plenty of excess fat rolled around our bellies, thighs, and arms: 20 pounds, 25, 30, 40, 50, 60, 75 and more! Your weight-bearing joints, especially the knees and hips, must struggle to support the useless, burdensome weight. And that is stress!

Start your offensive against arthritis by stepping on your scale. Obesity worsens arthritic conditions. Losing weight will not cure arthritis but it will take quite a burden off your overworked joints. This is not a diet book, so I will not discuss weight loss in great detail. If you are obese, read my earlier book, *the Beverly Hills* Medical *Diet*.

## OVERWEIGHT VERSUS OBESITY

To be overweight means to weigh more than the average person with your body build and height. Being overweight is not necessarily bad. For example, weight lifters and football players weigh more than the average person with their body size, but their extra weight is made up of muscle, not fat.

Obesity is not the same as overweight. You can be skinny *and* obese at the same time. Overweight refers to pounds—obesity is a measure of body fat. Many of the fashion models I see in my office are very skinny: 100, 110 pounds. But they have a high percentage of body fat—as much as 30 percent of their weight is accounted for by pure fat. It is the *percent of body fat* that determines if you are obese, not your absolute weight.

The simplest way to get a relatively accurate measure of your body fat is to ask your doctor for a skin caliper measurement of body fat. This is a fast and absolutely painless method of determining your ratio of body fat to lean body tissue (muscles, bones, organs, etc.) What looks like a pair of pliers with a meter build into it is used to "pinch the fat" at different points on your body. The meter measurements are used to figure out what percent of your body is made up of fat.

You need a certain amount of fat. Fat cushions organs, stores energy, provides a medium for vital fat-soluble chemicals, and has other functions. But too much fat is a killer. Too much fat causes or worsens just about every major disease, and it is strongly linked to heart disease, stroke, and cancer. Here are *my* general body fat guidelines for adults:

- Women should have about 20–25 percent body fat.
- Men should have about 10–12 percent body fat.
- Athletic women should have about 18–20 percent body fat
- Athletic men should have about 8–10 percent body fat.

(These figures do not apply to pregnant or lactating women, children, professional or "serious" athletes.)

## WEIGHT-LOSS SECRET

Calories in minus calories out-equals weight loss or gain. That is the weight-loss secret.

No, I am not being facetious. If you take in (eat) more calories than you expend you will gain weight. If you burn off more calories than you ingest you will lose weight. Many of my patients have told me that they have a metabolic condition that prevents them from losing weight. Only a very tiny percentage of people have a physical problem that prevents them from losing weight. For most people, it's a matter of eating too many calories. This is a weight-loss affirmation I have my patients say before they eat. It reminds them of their goal—cutting back the number of calories they eat:

I love my body and thank it for serving me well, now and in the future. Right now I give my physical being, *my body,* permission to weigh (*fill in your desired weight*). I deserve to be beautiful: physically, emotionally, and spiritually. The power of my love for myself and for life gives me the strength to handle my desires. I am now open to receiving all the blessings of this abundant universe.*

I have my patients say this before they eat. It really works!

## VEGGIE-BAGGIE

Leave gourmandizing; know the grave doth gape
For thee thrice wider than for other men.

Shakespeare, *Henry IV*

I have all my patients carry a baggie full of fresh green vegetables with them all day. Movie star, lawyer, housewife, student, retired person; I want them all to fill their baggie with fresh green vegetables for munching on during the day. Carrying your veggie-baggie is a good idea because:

1. You never have to look around for nutritious food to eat.
2. Vegetables are full of complex-carbohydrates, fiber, vitamins, and minerals.
3. You're never hungry because your baggie-veggies are always right at hand.
4. You have a constant reminder of what you should be eating to lose weight and gain health.

The baggie-veggies are part of my high complex carbohydrate Antistress Diet. Eat plenty of fresh vegetables because they help you get rid of those excess pounds. Vegetables are low-calorie, high-nutrition packets of health.

---

*If you want a copy of this affirmation on a card you can carry with you, write to me enclosing a self-addressed stamped envelope:
Arnold Fox, M.D.
436 N. Roxbury Drive
Suite 212
Beverly Hills, CA 90210

## ALOE FOR ARTHRITIS

Aloe vera juice helps in the fight against arthritis by giving you vitamins, minerals, and other nutrients to build up your general health. I have my patients begin with 2 ounces of aloe vera juice mixed with fruit juice at breakfast, slowly building up to bowel tolerance (loose stools). This is the general schedule I give my patients.

**Day 1:**   2 oz. with breakfast
**Day 4:**   Add 2 oz. with lunch
**Day 7:**   Add 2 oz. with dinner

They are now taking 2 oz. three times a day. They continue with this dosage until:

**Day 15:**   Add 2 oz. to the breakfast dose
**Day 18:**   Add 2 oz. to the lunch dose
**Day 21:**   Add 2 oz. to the dinner dose

They are now taking 4 oz. three times a day. I encourage them to take more if they can. But if this dose causes loose stools, I have them back down to bowel tolerance level.

## ACE AGAINST ARTHRITIS

ACE forms the base of the antiarthritis supplementation program I put most of my arthritis patients on. *ACE* stands for vitamins A, C, and E. Individual needs vary, and I cannot prescribe vitamins and minerals without first examining a patient. This is the general regimen I have most of my arthritic patients on:

VITAMIN A—10,000 IU of vitamin A, *plus* plenty of beta-carotene from vegetables and fruits. For beta-carotene eat two or three carrots a day, plus green and orange vegetables and orange fruits often.

**B VITAMINS**—I suggest to my patients a B-complex vitamin containing 50 milligrams of the major B vitamins. I have them take one tablet, twice a day. In addition to the B complex, I recommend to my patients:

**NIACIN**—25 mg, three times a day. (Niacin is a form of vitamin $B_3$.) Gradually increase the dose to 100 mg, three times a day. If an unpleasant flush develops on the face or body, reduce the dosage until the flush disappears. Niacin seems to decrease joint stiffness and the deformity associated with arthritis.

**NIACINAMIDE**—for very severe cases of arthritis, 500 mg three times a day. Niacinamide is also a form of vitamin $B_3$, but does not cause a flush.

**VITAMIN $B_5$**—500 mg twice a day, once after breakfast and once after lunch. During an arthritis flareup the dosage is doubled to two 500 mg tablets after breakfast and two 500 mg tablets after lunch.

**VITAMIN C**—As with vitamin A, I have my patients taking two kinds of vitamin C. First is a buffered vitamin C powder, a hypoallergenic formula that contains the following in 1 teaspoon:

| | |
|---|---|
| Vitamin C | 2,350 mg |
| Calcium | 450 mg |
| Magnesium | 250 mg |
| Potassium | 99 mg |

With this buffered form of vitamin C (pH 6.3) the side effects sometimes seen with regular vitamin C are avoided. I have my patients take 1 teaspoon in a glass of water or juice with breakfast.

*In addition,* I have them take a 1,000 mg vitamin C in tablet form, three times a day, with meals. If they are enjoying at least a 50% improvement and feeling good at the end of four weeks, I have them stick with this dosage. If not, I usually have them take 2,000 mg three times a day, with meals.

**VITAMIN E**—400 mg of D-alpha tocopherol (vitamin E) twice a day, once after breakfast and once after lunch. I prefer the water-soluble form, available as a dry powder in a soft gelatin capsule. Vitamin E is an antioxidant which some authorities suggest slows the rate of aging, and does seem to slow the formation of arthritis.

**MINERALS**—I have my patients begin with a multiple mineral that contains one-quarter of the recommended daily allowance (RDA) for all the minerals, and take four tablets a day. In addition to the multimineral, I suggest to my patients:

**SELENIUM**—200 mcgm a day. Selenium is a potent free radical quencher and an antiaging ally of vitamin E.

**ZINC**—220 mg of zinc sulfate (50 mg of elemental zinc) a day, twice a day during an arthritis flare up.

I vary this plan according to an individual patient's needs, giving more or less as is indicated. When the DLPA Antiarthritis Plan has helped my patients to feel really good, I have them reduce their vitamin and mineral supplements, step by step, back down to the basic supplementation plan outlined in chapter 3.

## SEEING JOINTS MOVE

While you are losing weight and improving your general health with diet, aloe vera, vitamins and minerals, put the power of your mind into play. Begin to see your pain go away. Sit down in a quiet, comfortable room. Tell everyone you do not want to be disturbed for 20 minutes. Let's say your arthritis is in your hands. Look at your hands. Study them. Turn them over. Examine them from every possible angle. Concentrate on how your hands feel. Where is the pain? What kind of pain is it? Big pain, little pain? Steady, or intermittent pain? Does it always hurt, or only when you move? Does it feel like someone is cutting your hand? Burning your hand on the inside? Are there sharp little nails inside the joint(s)?

Lay your hands on your lap and close your eyes. Picture your hands in your mind's eye. See them not as they are, but as they will be: Healthy. Imagine yourself moving the fingers. Not too fast, take it easy. Slowly move one finger, then the next, the next, until all of them have been bent and flexed. Close your hands into fists. Squeeze the fists, gently at first, adding strength slowly. Then let them relax for a few moments. Move the fingers again, one at a time, a little faster than last time, with more power. Now make a strong fist. Open and close your fists, feeling their power and flexibility. Now imagine those hands to be writing or typing, playing the piano, opening cans, knitting—whatever you do.

Do this for 20 minutes at a time, three times a day. Seeing with your mind's eye what you want to happen is a big step toward making it happen.

## MAKING YOUR JOINTS MOVE

This is one of the antiarthritis affirmations I ask my patients to say 10, 20 times a day. Say it to yourself, say it out loud, say it all day long, in your home, in your car, at work—anytime in any place.

I give myself permission to feel healthy!
I allow my hands (or appropriate joints) to be strong and supple.
I allow my hands to move freely.
I allow my hands to feel great!

## KEEPING YOUR JOINTS FLEXIBLE

To diet, aloe, vitamins and minerals, visualization, and affirmations, add exercise. The PA Walking I discussed in chapter 3 is an excellent exercise. The point of PA Walking is to exercise to the best of your ability—not to set records. Some of my patients have such severe arthritis that almost any kind of exercise is too difficult for them. I have these patients do a series of chair exercises. For example:

ARM RAISES—sitting in a chair, place your hands on your lap. Raise your arms in front of you until they are straight up in the air (or as high as you can go). Lower your arms until your hands are back on your lap. Practice until you are able to do this 10 times without stopping. To make it more difficult, try holding a book in each hand while you do this exercise. The more weight you add the better. But don't overdo it.

Now let your arms hang free at your sides. Raise them to the sides, until they are straight up in the air (or as high as you can). Lower them and repeat. Practice until you can do this exercise 10 times without stopping. If you can add weight (by holding a book), do so.

ARM CIRCLES—sitting in a chair, extend your arms to the side at shoulder level. Move your arms forward, down, back, then return to the starting position. Make small circles with your arms in this way, gradually increasing the size of the circles. Now swing your arms in the opposite direction, starting with small circles and building to big circles. Practice until you can make circles without stopping for one minute.

SIDE TWIST—sitting in an armless chair, carefully twist your upper body to the right, then to the left. Start slowly, twisting as far as you can comfortably go to the right, left, right, left, and so on. Practice until you can do this for 30 seconds without stopping. You will find yourself twisting further as you continue practicing.

TOE TOUCHES—sitting on a chair, carefully lean forward, dropping your chest onto your lap. Don't pitch forward; *slowly* lower your chest down to your lap. Resting your chest on your lap, reach down and touch your toes with your hands. Grab onto your shoes and gently pull yourself further down. This exercise stretches your back. Be very careful when doing this. Make sure to maintain your balance at all times.

**LEG LIFTS**—While sitting, brace yourself by gripping the arms of your chair, or holding onto the front of the chair. Carefully raise your legs, knees bent, as high as you can. Lower and repeat. Practice until you can do this 10 times. Be very careful to maintain your balance in the chair. When you have mastered this exercise, increase the difficulty by holding your knees in the air for a count of 10 before lowering them. You can also do this exercise with extended legs.

**NECK ROLLS**—sitting in a chair, drop your chin to your chest. Roll your head to the right, back to the center, to the left, back to center, and so on. Do this a few times to warm up, then roll your head to the right, back, to the left, and back to the starting point. This is a complete neck roll. Practice the neck rolls until you can do 10 complete neck rolls in both directions.

These are just a few of the many exercises you can do in a chair. If you can't PA Walk, fine, exercise in your chair. You can exercise anytime, anywhere. All you need is a little imagination and determination.

## RELIEVING ARTHRITIS WITH DLPA

Now that all the health-building steps have been explained, let's look at DLPA. This is the basic schedule I start my arthritic patients on:

**375 Milligrams of DLPA Three Times a Day**

375 mg with breakfast
375 mg with lunch
375 mg with dinner

I instruct my patients to have regular meals: breakfast at 8 A.M., lunch at noon, and dinner between 5 and 6 P.M. in the evening. DL-phenylalanine should be taken with the meal, or within an hour after completing the meal. I prefer it to be taken five minutes after the meal.

On the third day, if no pain relief has occurred, I generally have them increase the dosage to:

**750 Milligrams of DLPA Three Times a Day**

750 mg with breakfast
750 mg with lunch
750 mg with dinner

If my patients have trouble sleeping at night because DLPA gives them a feeling of excitement or energy, I have them cut the dinner dose in half.

NOTE: *You do not have to stop taking any medication prescribed by your doctor to benefit from DLPA. In fact, DLPA can greatly enhance the effectiveness of aspirin and analgesic drugs.*

This is the basic plan, which I vary to meet the needs of individual patients. I carefully monitor their progress, adjusting the dosage up or down as needed.

*I tell my patients to stay with DLPA—give it a chance to work.*

My observation has been that it takes anywhere from two days to three weeks for DLPA to take effect. It may take as long as four to six weeks, so I encourage my patients not to get discouraged. DLPA is not fast acting like aspirin. It takes *at least* two days to have effect. Give it a chance to work!

When they have felt really good for a full week, I have my patients stop taking DLPA and wait for the symptoms to recur. They go on an alternating schedule, taking DLPA until they feel good for a full week, then not taking it until the symptoms reappear, and so on. Many of my patients only use DLPA one out of every three or four weeks. Patients are encouraged to adjust their dosage in consultation with their physician.

**DLPA and aspirin:** I have some of my patients taking DLPA and aspirin together. If they were already taking aspirin, I have them continue taking it while taking DLPA. The two work well together, enhancing each other's effectiveness.

CAUTION: *I recommend against using DLPA during pregnancy or lactation. Pregnant or lactating women should not expose the fetus or newborn to* anything *except their normal diet. It's best to be safe. Neither should any person suffering from the genetic disease phenyketonuria (PKU) take DLPA—they cannot metabolize phenylalanine normally. This also applies to those on a phenylalanine-restricted diet. Neither do I recommend the use of DLPA for children under the age of 14. I arbitrarily chose this age because as an internist and cardiologist I do not usually treat children. However, physicians experienced in treating children may wish to examine the DLPA literature. They may find an appropriate use for DLPA in children, such as juvenile rheumatoid arthritis.*

## ASPIRIN AND DLPA

In chapter 2, I pointed out that DLPA and aspirin together work well in controlling chronic pain. The same holds true for arthritis pain. The combination of DLPA and aspirin is probably the most effective treatment I have used to treat arthritis. Aspirin does have side effects, so it should not be used excessively. With the DLPA/aspirin combination you are taking less aspirin than you normally would. Thus, total aspirin consumption is generally low enough to avoid trouble. I prefer to have my patients use DLPA alone, but for more difficult cases I sometimes recommend DLPA and aspirin.

## DO NOT SELF-MEDICATE!

*Do not throw away the medicine(s) your doctor has prescribed for you. Do not alter the dosage or stop taking the medicine(s). Discuss DLPA and Dr. Fox's DLPA Program with your physician. A trained professional, your physician will be able to guide you through the intricacies of the human body and mind. The nice thing about DLPA is that it does not interfere with other medication. You do not need to stop taking your medicines to benefit from DLPA. You and your doctor can try DLPA without stopping your other medications. My experience with my patients has been that with DLPA I can carefully reduce my patient's other medicines, and often eliminate them entirely.*

## THE WHOLE IS GREATER THAN THE SUM OF THE PARTS

Remember, DLPA is a *part* of Dr. Fox's DLPA Antiarthritis Plan. Weight loss, the Antistress Diet, Mental Blueprints, PA Walking, and DLPA all have a role to play in building general health and fighting arthritis. DL-phenylalanine is a powerful weapon against arthritis when used as part of Dr. Fox's DLPA Antiarthritis Plan.

## PAIN FREE IN FOUR DAYS

After four months on Dr. Fox's DLPA Antiarthritis Plan, Edith, an 83-year-old woman, gave this report:

"My arthritis started 25 years ago in my knees. It wasn't very painful so I only took aspirin once in a while. Five years ago it spread to my shoulders, both my shoulders, and my hands. Then I fell down on my left elbow. Soon there was arthritis there. My doctor gave me aspirin and Tylenol with codeine, but I don't like to use that because it makes me feel sick. He gave me some other drugs. I don't remember their names. They made me feel sick so I stopped taking them.

"Then Dr. Fox gave me DLPA and the rest of his plan. Some of it sounded silly. We didn't have affirmations when I was a little girl. But Dr. Fox is such a nice man. He is so sincere. So I ate broccoli, and took vitamins, and said the affirmations, and took DLPA to make him happy.

"Four days later I woke up with *no pain*. And the swelling has gone down some in my hands and knees. I walked all around the house that day, and the next day I walked to my friend's house five blocks away. It was so nice to be able to walk again. Dr. Fox's Plan and DLPA worked. I feel good. I don't know if it's the affirmations, the broccoli, or the DLPA that make me feel better, so I do everything Dr. Fox says to do. And I bought an Olympics T-shirt to wear when I PA Walk."

# 8

# PREMENSTRUAL SYNDROME: MONTHLY MISERY

"I'm a corporate lawyer, Dr. Fox. I have to project a certain image—intelligent, cool, steadfast. Projecting that image is usually not difficult because I *am* intelligent, cool, steadfast. Most of the time. Five or six days a month I shake inside like a bowl of Jell-o. Outside the cool lawyer, inside I'm a wreck. I seem to radiate angriness. I end up screaming at everyone, even if they tiptoe around me. I have a nice trim figure. My clothes fit me beautifully, then suddenly I'm uncomfortable in them and my stomach sticks out and I feel miserably bloated. It's absolute misery, this bloated lady screaming at everyone."

That's how this 35-year-old woman described her unhappy experiences with premenstrual syndrome (PMS), a condition that has attracted nationwide media attention. The estimates as to how many women are affected vary; as many as 40 million women in this country are PMS victims. Some women are slightly discomforted, others are utterly ruined.

Perhaps the most notorious case of PMS involved Sandie Smith, a 30-year-old London barmaid who stabbed and killed a female co-worker in 1979. Backed by expert testimony she claimed to be unable to control herself when in the throes of PMS. Ms. Smith was sentenced to 3 years probation on the condition she receive treatment for her PMS. Another British

"PMS defense" case involved Christine English, a 37-year-old woman who killed her lover in 1980. She was found guilty of manslaughter due to PMS-induced "diminished capacity."

Most women's reactions to PMS are not nearly that severe. Still, the "average" symptoms are enough to ruin many lives. In my practice I have seen a large variety of symptoms, including irritability, mood swings, spontaneous and unprovoked anger, tension, crying jags, excitability, headaches, feelings of helplessness and hopelessness, mild to profound depression, fatigue, weakness, lethargy, swelling and tenderness of the breasts, abdominal bloating, asthma, acne, water retention, weight gain, and increased appetite (especially for sweets, chocolate, salty foods, and alcohol). To combat these symptoms women take diuretics (water pills), nonsteroidal anti-inflammatory drugs, Fiorinal (an analgesic and muscle relaxant), Valium, Empirin, Empirin with codeine, and many other drugs. Pills provide some relief—at a price. For example, Anaprox, a popular pain pill, has these frequent side effects: gastrointestinal bleeding, nausea, heartburn, abdominal pain, diarrhea, headaches, dizziness, and heart palpitations.

## GOD'S WILL, OR HORMONES?

Many theories have been offered to explain why women suffer PMS. Some say PMS is due to a hormonal imbalance, some that an immune system disorder is responsible, others insist that it is God's will. Psychological, physiological, social, and religious arguments of all types have been proposed, but none has led to a successful treatment.

Probably the most popular theory at this time is championed by Dr. Katharine Dalton, the British gynecologist who testified on behalf of the "PMS defense." Dalton feels PMS is caused by a relative deficiency of progesterone, a sex hormone involved in the menstrual cycle.

## PROGESTERONE MEGADOSES: BLESSING OR CURSE?

More than 200 clinics specializing in progesterone therapy have sprung up in this country in the last couple of years. Along with perhaps 4,000 private physicians, these clinics are pumping women full of progesterone hormone—in some cases up to 4,000 milligrams a day! (Typical doses begin at 200 or 400 milligrams per day, often working their way much higher.) These megadoses expose women's bodies to 10, sometimes 100 times as much progesterone as naturally occurs in the bloodstream. In small doses progesterone is a useful PMS treatment for some women, but many gynecologists are now saying what I've been saying for years: Progesterone megadoses may be dangerous.

## NO LONG-TERM SAFETY STUDIES

Dr. Dalton says progesterone megadose therapy is safe. Is it? The possible long-term side effects of progesterone megadose therapy have not been studied. We have no idea what will happen over time to the lining of the uterus (endometrium). Neither do we know what influence progesterone megadoses will have on other hormones.

We do know what happened when estrogen, another sex hormone, was given in large doses. Premarin, a tablet made up of estrogens, has been used for years to treat menopausal symptoms and osteoporosis. If you look under Premarin in the *Physician's Desk Reference* (1983), you'll see this bold-face warning: "Estrogens Have Been Reported to Increase the Risk of Endometrial Carcinoma." It goes on to report that estrogenic therapy has these and other side effects: vomiting, cramps, cholestatic jaundice, headache, migraine, dizziness, depression, edemia, and loss of scalp hair. The large amount of estrogen in the early birth-control pills also cause many problems:

> I remember two women in their thirties I saw back in 1969. I was called in as a consultant to examine these women. The high doses of estrogen in their birth-control pills led to the formation of tiny blood clots in the arteries of their lungs. The arteries were gradually blocked which increased pressure in the lungs (pulmonary hypertension). This in turn caused heart failure, enlargement of the arteries in the neck, and swelling of the liver, abdomen, and legs. By the time I saw them, medicine had no hope to offer. These two women died within a few weeks of each other. Seeing two young women die from the same problem, so close in time, is scary—very scary.

## PROGESTERONE OR PLACEBO?

Is progesterone megadose therapy as good as they claim, or is the placebo effect responsible for a measure—perhaps a large measure—of its success? Unfortunately, there are but a few studies comparing progesterone to placebo. A study published in a 1979 issue of the *British Journal of Psychiatry*[1] found no significant difference between progesterone and placebo. (Some have criticized this study, saying the participants were not properly chosen.) A 1976 article published in *The Journal of Clinical Obstetrics and Gynecology*,[2] reported that progesterone was not an effective treatment for depression associated with PMS. (Some have criticized this study on the grounds that unreasonable claims were unfairly made for progesterone.)

What is the final word on progesterone megadose therapy? We don't know yet. Based on the evidence now available, I would not recommend the large progesterone dose presently used. We just don't know what will happen.

## DLPA: A SAFE AND EFFECTIVE ALTERNATIVE

Why run risks on progesterone megadose therapy when the Dr. Fox DLPA PMS Plan is a safe and effective alternative? Let Kathrine R. tell you her experience with the Plan:

"I've had PMS for seven years. I've spent one week every month getting traffic tickets, kicking my dog, fighting with my husband, looking for problems with clerks in stores, yelling at my kids. I was completely opposite to what I was like the rest of the time. You know what my son used to do? If someone asked him what the date was he would say 'two weeks past PMS!' Can you imagine what my PMS was doing to my family? My husband always forgave me, the kids understood, and the dog came crawling back, but I had to live with the memory of what I had done during my PMS. This went on for months, years!"

I asked Kathrine to go on my DLPA PMS Plan. She changed her eating habits and her outlook, and took DLPA as directed. Six months later she said: "It's amazing, Dr. Fox.

All the craziness is gone. It used to be that my period ran my life. Now I'm in control. And my son doesn't tell time by my PMS anymore."

## PMS: AN ENDORPHIN WITHDRAWAL?

Women describing their PMS often mention symptoms similar to the symptoms of narcotic withdrawal, such as severe abdominal cramps and restlessness. This raises a provocative question: Could PMS be caused by a temporary "withdrawal" from the internal opiates (endorphins)?

A link has been proposed between PMS and endorphins in articles published in 1981 in the *American Journal of Obstetrics and Gynecology*[3] and in *Medical Hypothesis*.[4] The connection is based on biochemical evidence indicating that endorphins interact with a number of female sex hormones.[5] Studies with experimental animals have found that the levels of brain endorphins fluctuate significantly over the course of the menstrual cycle.

Based on the present evidence, it is most likely that the PMS complex of symptoms could be at least partially due to a temporary deficiency of beta-endorphin and/or enkephalins in the brain. A variation of this idea is that there are enough endorphins present in the brain, but that the endorphin receptors are temporarily less sensitive (less likely to form a lock-and-key bond with endorphins).

The endorphins help regulate our pain threshold: If PMS is caused by a temporary endorphin withdrawal, wouldn't PMS sufferers experience more pain (lowered pain threshold)? In reviewing the PMS literature, I was struck by the wording in one of the first major medical reports of PMS.[6] This paper noted that a "lowered pain threshold" was one of the three major PMS symptoms. The authors of this paper pointed out that women complained that they "just can't stand pain."

My personal belief is that a decrease in endorphin levels is partially responsible for many of the symptoms of PMS. Continued study will hopefully give the medical community greater insight into the exact mechanisms by which DLPA helps relieve many PMS symptoms.

## PEA FOR PMS?

In chapter 4, I mentioned the link between PEA and depression. Are the mood changes seen with PMS related to fluctuating PEA levels? This is a reasonable supposition, but unfortunately, one that lacks solid corroborating evidence. If a change in PEA levels does trigger PMS mood shifts, then DLPA may owe some of its anti-PMS effects to its ability to raise PEA levels. I believe that future research will establish a firm link between PEA and PMS.

In the meantime, it's interesting to note that many women tend to crave chocolate, which contains relatively large amounts of PEA, before and during their menstrual period. Are the women unknowingly attempting to increase their PEA levels? In order to do so, they would have to consume very large quantities of chocolate, and so far, there is no evidence supporting the idea that chocolate is a cure for PMS (although it is a tasty try). I suggest to my PMS patients they forgo the chocolate and stick with my DLPA anti-PMS plan.

## TOO MANY OF THEM

While I was examining Greg, a 28-year-old construction worker, he told me that he was thinking of divorcing his wife.

"I love my wife," he said. "I love her enough to put up with her being crazy four days a month. I mean, absolutely crazy. Screaming, crying, throwing things. I can live with that but I can't take the rest of them. I live right by my mother-in-law and her four sisters. But every so often they go crazy, crying, fighting with each other, and they start in with the yelling and screaming. I can put up with my wife, but not all six of them. It's been going on for eight years and I've had enough!"

The next week Greg brought his wife to see me. She responded very well to DLPA and my DLPA–PMS Plan. Greg is not thinking about a divorce anymore: He's trying to get his mother-in-law and her sisters onto the Plan.

# 9

# DR. FOX'S DLPA–PMS PLAN

"I can't really remember when PMS entered my life—it just came on gradually after the onset of menses. Looking back through the years I remember 'being crazy' on some days. I didn't pinpoint it to every month, it just suddenly came and just as suddenly left. PMS was like there was a woman—angry—screaming at her husband and children, while inside there was the usual calm woman looking at the screaming woman on the outside and wondering 'What is wrong with her? Why is she so mad?' It's like there are two people; the 'real you' and the 'PMS you.' PMS completely surrounds and swallows you. You can't get out, you can't protest; you can only wait until tomorrow or the next day when the real you is released. Then everyone you came in contact with during the PMS tiptoes around you, afraid of another outburst. You feel terrible, but apologies are useless. Everyone says 'That's all right, don't worry about it'; but you do. You wonder what emotional stress you are heaping upon your children and marriage. When my children were little a friend told me these 'days' occurred because of the onset of menses and it could be relieved a little by taking a water pill. So each month when PMS began I would take water pills. There was a lot of relief—for my family—because I was too busy in the bathroom to scream at them. It also relieved my waistline a bit. But as soon as I was out of the bathroom the anger and screaming continued."

Although I have known this woman for many, many years, it was only recently that I began to treat her for PMS. She resisted the Dr. Fox DLPA–PMS Plan at first—she wanted what she called "real medicine." But after talking with other women who are on my DLPA–PMS Plan she agreed to give it a try. Six months later she said:

> "I'm one again. It's no longer the 'real me' trapped inside the 'PMS me.' The 'PMS me' is gone. Forever. My family no longer has to tiptoe around me during my period. I wish I knew about this 20 years ago."

## FOUR-PRONGED ATTACK

You are already very familiar with the general outline and philosophy of my DLPA Program, so let's get right down to specifics: How to use the DLPA Program to fight PMS. We'll look at the four elements—the Antistress Diet, Mental Blueprints, PA Exercise, and DLPA—and how they contribute to the fight against PMS.

Remember, all four elements are necessary to beat PMS. No single part will do it. The Plan only works if you carefully build a foundation of excellent health topped off with DLPA.

## SSPC: STOP *SICKENING PREMENSTRUAL CYCLES*

I tell my patients that to stop PMS they must SSPC: *S*top *S*ickening *P*remenstrual *C*ycles by eliminating *s*alt, *s*ugar, *p*rocessed foods, and *c*affeine from their diet. SSPC: *S*alt, *S*ugar, *P*rocessed foods, and *C*affeine.

These food stuffs have been implicated in high blood pressure, heart disease, stroke, cancer, diabetes, irregular heart rhythms, kidney disease, vision loss, and many other problems, including PMS.

## SALT: BLOATING IS JUST THE BEGINNING

Do you know how much salt you eat every day? I ask my patients to write down everything they have eaten for the past several weeks, then use a computer to estimate their daily salt intake (among other things). People who never add salt to their food are amazed to find out how much salt they consume. There is salt everywhere, hidden in places you would not suspect. Did you know that Alka-seltzer has over 500 mg of sodium per tablet and Bromo seltzer has over 700 mg of sodium per tablet?

Let's say you eat a frozen chicken dinner one evening. You do not add any salt, but it already has about 1,100 milligrams of sodium added by the food manufacturer. With your chicken you have a canned soup. Canned soup has about 1,100 milligrams of sodium in it, too. You have a glass of milk with your dinner; that's another 50 milligrams of sodium. Half an hour later your stomach is upset, so you take two Alka-seltzers—another 1,000 milligrams of sodium.

You haven't touched the salt shaker, but you've already swallowed *over 3,200 milligrams of sodium* in one meal!

Adults only need an average of about 400 milligrams of sodium a day to keep their body's metabolic machinery in good shape. Table salt is 40 percent sodium, so it only takes about one-twentieth of a teaspoon of table salt to fulfill your daily requirement. You need some sodium because it's involved with regulating the amount of water in your body. Your body's fluids must have a certain "saltiness." If the fluids become too "salty," the body triggers water-retaining mechanisms that keep more water in the body to water down the salt. Meanwhile, the kidneys are working hard to get rid of the excess sodium. In some situations, water will move out of your cells to help dilute the too-salty body fluids. That helps the fluids, but harms the cells.

Salt also causes arterioles (small arteries) to constrict. This can raise your blood pressure. Elevated blood pressure increases the risk of a break in your network of arteries. If this break occurs in the brain it may lead to a stroke.

Throwing off the sodium–fluid ratio is just one of the many problems associated with salt. To put it in a nutshell; salt is stress.

I have found that just getting women to cut back on the amount of salt they consume helps relieve PMS.

Stop adding salt to your food. Don't eat obviously salty foods, like pretzels, potato chips, salted nuts, and most other junk foods. Learn to look for hidden salts in food:

1. Any canned, packaged, frozen, or prepared food is liable to have lots of salt in it. Food processors love to put salt into their concoctions. Cake mixes are full of salt. So are commercial breads, cheese, butter, sandwich meats, mustard, commercial pizza, rolls and buns, salad dressings, sandwich spreads, canned or dehydrated soups. The general rule of thumb is this: If the food is man-made or processed it is probably loaded with added salt, so eat nature's food instead.

2. Learn to look for these salty ingredients:
   • Sodium chloride is table salt.
   • Sodium alganate is used in ice cream and chocolate drinks for a smoother texture.
   • Sodium benzoate is used by manufacturers as a food preservative.
   • Sodium hydroxide is considered a poison in the chemistry laboratory. But believe it or not, it is used to process ripe olives, hominy, and some fruits and vegetables.
   • Sodium sulfite is sprayed on lettuce and salads to make them look fresh. Many people are severely allergic to this substance.
   • Sodium propionate is often added to some breads, cakes, and pasteurized cheese.
   • Disodium phosphate is in some quick-cooking cereals and in processed cheeses. Watch out for it.
   • Monosodium glutamate (MSG) is found as a seasoning, especially in Chinese restaurants. When dining at a Chinese restaurant ask your waiter to ask the cook to leave salt and MSG out of your food.
   • Baking soda (sodium bicarbonate) is used to make cakes, breads, and other bakery goods. It is often added to vegetables as they are cooked. People also take baking soda for indigestion.
   • Baking powder is found in breads, cakes, pastries.
   • Brine contains a lot of sodium. Watch out for brine in

pickles, pickled foods, and many canned, processed, and frozen foods.

Read food labels carefully. Watch out for *any* mention of sodium.


## AVOID, AVOID, AVOID

These are some of the sodium-rich foods I tell my patients to avoid:

Anchovies
Bacon
Bacon fat
Bouillon cubes (use the salt-free ones)
Catsup (use the salt-and sugar-free brands)
Caviar
Cheese (use sodium-free cheese)
Chili sauce (use sodium-free brands)
Chipped beef
Corned beef
Garlic salt (use fresh garlic or garlic powder instead)
Herring
Hot dogs
Luncheon meats
Meat sauces
Meat tenderizers
Mustard (get the brands without salt)
Olives
Onion salt (use fresh onions)
Pickles (full of salt!)
Salted popcorn (unsalted popcorn tastes good and is good for you)
Potato chips (really a bunch of fat covered with salt)
Pretzels
Relishes
Salt (throw away your salt shaker)
Salted and smoked meats
Salted pork

Salted and smoked fish
Sardines
Sauerkraut
Soy sauce (occasionally using reduced-salt soy sauce is okay)

I don't mean you should never eat salt or salty foods: just keep it to an absolute minimum. Here are a few figures to give you an idea of how much sodium you may be unknowingly eating.

|  |  | *Approximate milligrams of sodium* |
|---|---|---|
| Ham (cured) | 3 ounces | 675 |
| Hot dog | one regular | 540 |
| Bologna | one slice | 390 |
| Chicken | 3 ounces | 75 |
| Beef | 3 ounces | 75 |
| Veal | 3 ounces | 75 |
| Lamb | 3 ounces | 75 |
| Pork (not cured) | 3 ounces | 75 |
| Egg | one | 60 |

And some comparisons:

| | | |
|---|---|---|
| Salted nuts | ¼ cup | 275 |
| Unsalted nuts | ¼ cup | 2 |
| | | |
| Corn flakes | 1 cup | 165 |
| Shredded wheat | 1 cup | 1 |
| Puffed wheat | 1 cup | 1 |
| | | |
| Salted margarine | 1 tablespoon | 110 |
| Unsalted margarine | 1 tablespoon | 1 |
| | | |
| Creamed cottage cheese | ¼ cup | 160 |
| Unsalted cottage cheese | ¼ cup | 30 |
| | | |
| American, cheddar, Swiss, and Muenster cheese | 1 ounce | 220 |
| Parmesan cheese | 1 ounce | 80 |

Nature puts as much sodium in your food as you need. But man turns this fine, natural item, sodium, into a killer by dumping huge amounts of it into foods. Stick with fresh, natural foods. The food companies will not be happy, but your body will.

## MORE ON THE SUGAR DRAGON

What is the difference between sugar, dextrose, and corn syrup? Answer: Not very much. Sugar, like salt, has many names. The sugar industry will tell you there is a difference, but as far as your body is concerned, there is no difference. They are all sugar, they all hit your body with the Sugar Dragon.

The Sugar Dragon is a strong, fiery burst of energy that blazes gloriously for a brief time. But you are left a burned out wreck when the Sugar Dragon retreats back into his cave.

Just a quick digression to remind you of the difference between complex carbohydrates and refined carbohydrates. Complex carbohydrates are long, tightly bound chains of individual glucose (sugar) units, while refined carbohydrates are short, loosely bound chains. The more refined the carbohydrate, the quicker it is broken down and sent into action. In case of dietary sugar, however, quick action can be hazardous to your health. Instead of getting too much energy too fast to handle, your body prefers a slow, steady entry of sugar into the bloodstream.

Refined carbohydrates are carbohydrates that have been subjected to different processing techniques. All the nutrition is stripped away from the complex carbohydrate foods, leaving only simple sugars. Take table sugar, for example. As a part of the sugar cane, sugar is found in association with fiber, vitamins, and minerals. To turn sugar cane into table sugar, you throw away all the fiber, vitamins, and minerals. As part of the sugar cane, sugar is not bad. By itself, sugar is poison.

Stay away from refined carbohydrates in the form of white bread, cakes, pies, pastries, pasta made from white flour, candy and other foods. Eat the complex carbohydrates found in vegetables, fruits, whole grains and legumes (peas, beans and lentils).

Remember the man I described in chapter 4, who suddenly became supercharged with energy after eating a piece of pie and a Coke? I measured his blood sugar every half an hour and plotted it on a graph. Here is a very striking visual "diagram" of what his body was suffering through:

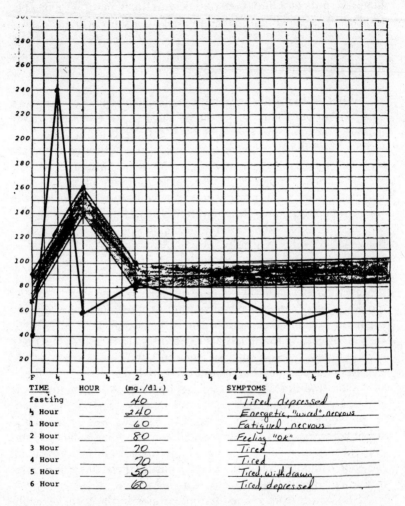

| TIME | HOUR | (mg./dl.) | SYMPTOMS |
|------|------|-----------|----------|
| fasting | ____ | 40 | Tired, depressed |
| ½ Hour | ____ | 240 | Energetic, "wired", nervous |
| 1 Hour | ____ | 60 | Fatigued, nervous |
| 2 Hour | ____ | 80 | Feeling "OK" |
| 3 Hour | ____ | 70 | Tired |
| 4 Hour | ____ | 70 | Tired |
| 5 Hour | ____ | 50 | Tired, withdrawn |
| 6 Hour | ____ | 60 | Tired, depressed |

The shaded area shows the route a person's blood sugar should follow after eating. It should go up, not too high, then smoothly drop to normal. The shaded area is wide enough to allow for individual variations.

This man started with a very low blood sugar. He ate the pie and coke, his blood sugar shot sky high, and the Sugar Dragon came stomping out. Then the Sugar Dragon left and the man came crashing down. Look how his blood sugar plummeted to way below normal. Now the man was tired, irritable, depressed. And look how his blood sugar went up and down, always missing the normal range, until it finally straightened itself out—*five hours later!*

All that time his blood sugar was bouncing up and down he felt terrible.

What do you think happens to a woman with PMS when she takes on the Sugar Dragon? You know who the loser is going to be. Sugar worsens the symptoms of PMS. Sugar creates stress.

I tell my PMS patients to avoid sugar, candy, ice cream, cake, pie, sodas, pastries, processed foods, canned foods, and other sugary foods. What should you eat instead? The Dr. Fox Antistress Diet: fresh vegetables and fruits, whole grains, peas, beans, and lentils, with small amounts of fish, poultry, and dairy products. Nature has put just as much sugar in these foods as you need for the best of health.

## PROCESSED FOODS: SLOW STRANGULATION

A supermarket may have as many as 10,000 items on its shelves. But the various packaged and processed foods are filled with fat, sugar, salt, coloring, flavoring, texturizers, and other chemicals. These ubiquitous processed foods are slowly but surely strangling our health.

Let's take breakfast cereals as an example. Starting off your day with cereal (real cereal) is great. You get lots of complex carbohydrates, vitamins, minerals, fiber, and small amounts of fat and protein.

But instead of natural, whole grain cereals, we gobble up processed cereals like Captain Crunch, Frankenberry, Strawberry Shortcake, Coco Puffs, Rice Krispies, and Pac Man cereal. Just looking at Frankenberry's ingredients is enought to frighten me because this cereal is nothing but sugar, salt, fat, texturizers, flavorers, preservatives, and chemicals–a bowl full of stress!

Most of the rest of the processed foods on supermarket shelves are not much healthier. Stick with fresh fruits, fresh vegetables, and whole grains. Leave the processed foods alone!

## CAFFEINE: JITTERY MISERY

Is it possible for you to have a sugar reaction, even if you did not eat sugar? Yes. Caffeine will do it to you. Caffeine stimulates your adrenal glands and other parts of your body. The adrenals release chemicals called catecholamines which prompt the liver to release stored sugar into the bloodstream. Your pancreas responds by sending out insulin to capture the Sugar Dragon and your blood sugar level comes crashing down. You feel tired, irritable, depressed. It's a sugarlike reaction without the sugar.

Besides uncaging the Sugar Dragon, caffeine stimulates your heart and muscles, irritates the lining of your stomach, leads to an increase in stomach acid, and encourages heartburn.

The net effect is stress and a consequent worsening of PMS symptoms.

## ARMED AGAINST PMS WITH VITAMINS AND MINERALS

I tell my PMS patients to take the basic vitamin and mineral regimen described in chapter 3 until they are midway through their mentrual cycle. Halfway between their menstrual periods (which is midcycle) I have them switch to this vitamin and mineral schedule:

VITAMIN A—Eat two or three carrots a day to get plenty of beta-carotene. Also eat lots of orange and green vegetables, and orange fruits.

B COMPLEX—A hypoallergenic B-complex tablet containing 50 mg of the major B vitamins plus 400 mcgm of folic acid. Take one three times a day.

VITAMIN $B_6$   200 mg three times a day.

VITAMIN C   One teaspoon buffered vitamin C powder in water or juice with breakfast, *plus* one 1,000 mg tablet after each meal. (Three times a day.)

**VITAMIN E** 400 IU D-alpha tocopherol (vitamin E) twice daily

**CALCIUM CARBONATE** 1,000 mg with 400 of vitamin D. Take right before bed.

**IRON** 1 Vitron-C tablet daily. It is available at your pharmacy without a prescription.

**MAGNESIUM** 400 mg tablet of elemental magnesium three times a day, with meals.

**ZINC SULFATE** Take 220 mg once a day, with breakfast.

**TRYPTOPHAN**—1 500 mg capsule of this amino acid after breakfast, another 500 mg after dinner. If necessary, this can slowly be increased to six capsules a day, three in the morning, and three in the evening.

If PMS symptoms are very severe, I ask my patients to add:

**EVENING PRIMROSE OIL**—Evening Primrose Oil is rich in linoleic acid, an essential fatty acid. This oil is needed for the production in your body of a prostaglandin known as PGE[1]. PGE seems to play a role in the reduction of some PMS symptoms. I have my patients take two capsules twice a day before menses. This may be increased to three times a day before menses if necessary. If Evening Primrose Oil does not help within two menstrual cycles, I have my patients discontinue its use.

This is the basic plan, which I vary according to the needs of my individual patients. When the DLPA–PMS Plan has helped my patients to feel really good, I have them reduce their supplementation, step by step, back down to the basic supplementation outlined in chapter 3.

## ALOE FOR PMS

I also have my PMS patients drinking aloe vera juice because aloe is an excellent general tonic, and it is therefore good for general health, which in turn helps fight PMS. I have them start with 2 ounces a day, slowly building up to 4 ounces, three times a day (for a total of 12 ounces a day). The general guideline I give them is to take as much as they can up to bowel tolerance (loose stools).

For the exact dosage schedule I recommend for my patients see chapter 3.

## "I CHOOSE"

"Choose," I tell my PMS patients. "Choose strong Mental Blueprints." Depression is a major problem with PMS. Write your positive Mental Blueprints now, before PMS, so you are ready. Premenstrual syndrome affirmations do not have to deal with PMS directly; they may be of a more general, but always very positive, nature. Here is one I give my patients:

> I love my body.
> I lovingly care for my body.
> I choose health and happiness.
> I choose to live the good life,
> Inspired by my thoughts of health
> and happiness.
> What I choose in my heart and
> mind, I choose for my life.
> I choose the best for myself!

## PA AEROBICS

In the last decade or so, more and more women have begun to exercise. The marvelous results are clear to all. In the last five years especially, I have seen a lot of women who do aerobic exercising or aerobic dancing. Aerobics are especially helpful for

PMS sufferers because the classes emphasize strengthening stomach and back muscles.

PMS sufferers often complain of stomach and back pains. Building up those muscles is an excellent way to head off cramps and back pain. I recommend to my PMS patients they select an aerobics class that:

1. is neither too advanced nor too slow for them;
2. works on strengthening stomach and back muscles;
3. does not neglect the heart (includes at least 20 minutes of running in place, jumping, bouncing, or other exercises that get the heart beating at 70 to 80 percent of its maximal rate); and
4. is fun!

Aerobics are great! They get you moving, stretching, building, and firming, and they are fun. But be careful. Don't overdo it at first, and make sure that your feet and the floor are properly padded so you do not stress your feet and knees.

Add Positive Affirmations (PA) to your aerobics and you will be working on mind and body together. Positive Affirmation Walking, PA Jogging, PA Swimming, and other PA aerobic exercises are also good for your Mental Blueprints and your health.

## DLPA FOR PMS

DL-phenylalanine for PMS is just a little tricky because unlike chronic pain and depression, PMS comes and goes. That makes it more difficult to fine tune the dosage. I have my patients who weigh more than 110 pounds start with:

**375 milligrams of DLPA twice a day:**

375 mg with breakfast
375 mg with lunch

If this dosage level does not produce the desired results, I generally have them increase their dosage to:

**375 milligrams of DLPA three times a day:**

375 mg with breakfast
375 mg with lunch
375 mg with dinner

I have my patients begin on this schedule four to seven days before their PMS symptoms are expected, and stop taking DLPA at the end of menses, or when their symptoms disappear.

I also instruct my patients to have regular meals: breakfast at 8:00 A.M., lunch at noon, and dinner between 5 and 6 P.M. DL-phenylalanine should be taken with the meal, or within an hour after completing the meal. I prefer it to be taken five minutes after the meal.

NOTE: *You do not have to stop taking any medication prescribed by your doctor to benefit from DLPA. In fact, DLPA may greatly enhance the effectiveness of other PMS treatments.*

This is the basic plan, which I vary to meet the needs of individual patients. I carefully monitor their progress, adjusting the dosage up or down as needed.

*I tell my patients to stay with DLPA—give it a chance to work.* My patients begin taking DLPA four to seven days before their PMS episode is expected to begin. They continue taking it on through their menses. Starting on DLPA at this time will begin to raise endorphin levels gradually so that symptoms generally do not occur. You do not have to take DLPA when your menstrual period is over. Working together, you and your physician will be able to determine the best time for you to start taking DLPA.

CAUTION: *I recommend against using DLPA during pregnancy or lactation. Pregnant or lactating women should not expose the fetus or newborn to* anything *except their normal diet. It's best to be safe. Neither should any person suffering from the genetic disease phenylketonuria (PKU) take DLPA—they cannot metabolize phenylalanine normally. This also applies to those on a phenylalanine-restricted diet. Neither do I recommend the use of DLPA for children under the age of 14. I arbitrarily chose this age because as an internist and cardiologist I do not usually treat children. Physicians experienced in treating children may wish to examine the DLPA literature. They may find an appropriate use for DLPA in children, such as juvenile rheumatoid arthritis.*

## PMS PLAN WRAP-UP

A fist is most effective when all the fingers work together. Think of all the parts of Dr. Fox's DLPA–PMS Plan—the Anti-stress Diet, Mental Blueprints, PA Exercise, and DLPA—as the fingers making up the fist that will knock out your PMS. *All* the fingers are important.

Give PMS the one-two punch with your strongest fist—use the entire DLPA–PMS Plan.

## DO NOT SELF-MEDICATE!

*But remember: Self-medication can be dangerous. Do not throw away or stop taking the medicine(s) your doctor has prescribed for you. Discuss DLPA and Dr. Fox's DLPA Program with your physician. A trained professional, your physician will be able to guide you through the intricacies of the human mind and body. The nice thing about DLPA is that it does not interfere with other medications. You do not need to stop taking other medications to benefit from DLPA. You and your doctor can try DLPA without stopping your other medication. My experience with my patients has been that with DLPA I can carefully reduce my patient's other medicine, and often eliminate it entirely.*

## PMS, NOT DRUGS

Diane was a 15-year-old girl brought to me by her mother. Although not a good student, Diane was bright, well read, and very articulate. She was about 15 pounds overweight and had a moderate amount of teenage acne, but was otherwise in good health. Her diet was the usual teenage grab bag of junk: burgers, pizza, soda, candy. Her mother told me that Diane was having problems in school; her grades were low and the teachers reported that sometimes she became angry and flighty. They suspected she was on drugs.

"She's not on drugs, Dr. Fox. I'm her mother. I can tell. Diane is a sweet, loving, caring, and all around wonderful girl. Most of the time. Please. Help her."

When I began explaining to Diane why what she was eating was bad for her, she starting lecturing me on physiology and chemistry! She knew stuff I did not hear of until I got to medical school. With her background and enthusiasm, she quickly understood why my DLPA PMS Plan would help her and agreed to go on the Plan.

What a wonderful patient! She called every morning to give me a full report on what she ate the day before, how much she exercised, and what her impressions were. She even composed her own affirmations. In no time at all her PMS was a thing of the past.

## "I LOVE DLPA AND NEVER WANT TO BE WITHOUT IT"

A woman in her late twenties was so dramatically affected by PMS she described herself as "having the loveable personality of an ax murderess" two weeks of every month. Ten days to two weeks before her periods her back started hurting, her belly bloated, the texture of her skin changed, she became irritable and depressed. Completely incapacitated, she could only lie in bed, curled up in a ball, for several days. Aspirin, Pamprin, Midol, and similar over-the-counter remedies only provided "about 10 percent relief." She mistrusted and was allergic to many prescription drugs.

She began the DLPA Program about six days before she expected her PMS symptoms to begin one month—and experienced "about 80 percent relief!" The second month she waited until only two days before her symptoms were due to take DLPA. Still, she enjoyed "90 to 100 percent relief. A complete change in my life!"

She continued successfully on the program for eight months, then decided to see what would happen if she stopped. The first month off the Plan was all right. Apparently DLPA's effects carried over from the previous month. But the second month, all of her old PMS symptoms returned in full force.

"That's enough testing," she said, and went back on the DLPA Plan. Two years have passed, and all of her symptoms have subsided, leaving her fully functional for the first time in many years. She reports increased energy and an overall sense of well-being. "It's changed my life. It's an ideal treatment. I love DLPA and never want to be without it!"

## "A WAR ZONE"

Marsha's mother died when she was six. There were no close family members to help raise Marsha, so her father put her in a convent school. Marsha stayed at the convent many years, seeing her father only at Christmas. When she was 16 she demanded to live with him in Los Angeles and moved into his apartment, which soon became what he described as a "war zone."

The father did not know how to handle children, especially a child he had had little contact with for 10 years. On top of that, he had a lot of guilt feelings; in the back of his mind he felt he had abandoned her. As if that were not enough, Marsha had severe PMS. Every month they had a week-long knock down, drag-em-out fight, with neighbors complaining about the yelling and the maid complaining about the broken dishes and vases. Her father was convinced Marsha was mentally deranged, a Jekyll and Hyde. He asked me to examine her.

I examined Marsha, then we spoke for 2 hours. Yes, she harbored resentment against her father for "dumping me in the convent." But she was willing to forgive him. As soon as Marsha forgave her father her PMS problems were cut in half! The anger she carried inside her all those years had made her PMS much worse than it had to be. Letting go of that anger helped her quite a bit. I also got her to change her eating habits and join an aerobic dancing class.

You know what? She never took DLPA. She didn't have to. Letting go of her anger, eating properly, and exercising was all it took to get rid of her PMS. She found out what a wonderful lot of good a little bit of forgiveness can do.

# 10

# SHARPENING ACUPUNCTURE WITH DLPA

Acupuncture, the ancient Chinese medical technique, has been used in Asia to treat various diseases and painful conditions for at least 4,500 years. American surgeons were stunned in the early 1970s as they watched Chinese surgeons performing major operations on patients—without anesthetics. Photographs were printed in many American medical journals, showing smiling patients lying on operating tables, organs exposed, with acupuncture needles sticking out of their face or hands. Western medical science was, to say the least, skeptical and hostile to this intriguing method of controlling pain.

This attitude has changed, however, and today there are an estimated 2,000 physicians practicing acupuncture in this country and some American medical schools now offer acupuncture courses for continuing education credit.

Several impressive clinical trials have tested acupuncture's affect on pain. In 1973, a National Institutes of Health committee on acupuncture reported on studies involving more than 400 patients in eight pain clinics: 60 percent of the patients enjoyed good to excellent pain relief. In a 1974 study at Hahneman University, 60 percent of the 108 osteoarthritis patients experienced excellent to complete relief from their pain.

These and other studies were not universally accepted by the medical community, but they raised some very interesting questions. How does acupuncture work? American scientists dismissed Chinese explanations which rested on the existence of mysterious body energies, preferring a more scientific explanation.

More recently Chinese researchers performed an interesting experiment in which they found that you could transfer the effects of acupuncture from one animal to another! They used acupuncture to block one animal's pain, they took some blood or spinal fluid from that animal and gave it to another animal that *had not* had acupuncture: The second animal's pain was also blocked! This strongly suggested that acupuncture triggered the release of some hormone or chemical, which could be transferred from one animal to another.

What was this substance? Dr. Daniel Mayer and his colleagues at the Medical College of Virginia thought that acupuncture might somehow trigger the release of endorphins in the body.[1] They tested this idea in 1976 using two groups of subjects. Each group was given acupuncture. Group 1 then received an injection of naloxone, the endorphin blocker; group 2 was injected with water (neither group knew what was in their injection). Both groups were then subjected to tooth shock. Naloxone *blocked* acupuncture's pain-relieving effects! Researchers concluded that the endorphins must be involved.

Other studies have supported the endorphin/acupuncture link. One report published in *The Lancet* (1980), a prominent medical journal, reported that acupuncture raised the levels of beta-endorphin in the spinal fluid of 10 patients.[2] In another study, spinal fluid samples from 12 patients who underwent abdominal surgery were collected before and after acupuncture.[3] Endorphins increased in 7 of the 12. Compare this to 4 patients who underwent the same surgical procedure, but did not have acupuncture. Their endorphin levels *decreased*.

Acupuncture seems to block pain by releasing endorphins, and DL-phenylalanine (DLPA) protects the endorphins. Would DLPA enhance the effects of acupuncture? Dr. Richard Cheng and Dr. Bruce Pomeranz at the University of Toronto found that DPA, along with several other compounds, increased the effectiveness of acupuncture in laboratory animals.[4] Naloxone, the endorphin blocker, reversed the effects.

Next was the test on human pain patients. A Japanese research team found that DPA strengthened acupuncture in patients with low back pain and patients undergoing dental surgery. In normal (nonpained) subjects, DPA increased their ability to withstand pain. Then the researchers gave D-phenylalanine (DPA) to patients who did not respond to acupuncture—with DPA they responded. The researchers noted:

> If any method such as DPA administration is discovered by which [acupuncture] analgesia or anesthesia is potentiated . . . [acupuncture] treatment would be further developed. This seems to be the case with DPA.[5]

More scientific study is needed, but all indications are that DLPA and DPA enhance the effects of acupuncture. Acupuncture therapists may soon ask their pain patients to prepare for acupuncture treatment by taking DLPA several days before their visits.

# 11

# WHAT ARE ENDORPHINS?

*Among the remedies which it has pleased Almighty God to give man to relieve his sufferings, none is so universal and efficacious as opium.*

—A 17TH-CENTURY PHYSICIAN

## GOD'S OWN MEDICINE

The relief of pain has been man's seemingly quixotic passion throughout the ages. Opium had long been considered the strongest weapon in the battle against pain. So great was man's reliance on opium that, at the turn of this century, the great physician Sir William Osler referred to it as "God's own medicine." In 1803 a German chemist named Friedrich Wilhelm Serturner had isolated the active factor in opium—morphine. That paved the way for the derivation of other powerful analgesic and mood-altering drugs from this plant.

## BRAIN RECEPTORS FOR MORPHINE?

How does morphine block pain? Why does one get a sense of euphoria when using morphine? How do such small amounts of morphine elicit such tremendous responses? Does morphine kill pain by acting on neurons (nerve cells) right at the site of the injury, in selected areas of the brain, or somewhere in between?

These are some of the questions modern neuroscientists explored while trying to solve the morphine mystery. The most important clue was this: Morphine's ability to kill pain depended on what part of the body it was injected into. When injected into very specific areas in the core of the brain, morphine was *1,000 times stronger* than if injected into non-brain areas (such as muscle). That meant there must be something in the brain especially sensitive to morphine, something that could "work with" morphine.

But what is that something? Neural receptors were a likely candidate. An intricate network of neurons spread throughout your body allows your central nervous system (brain and spinal cord) to communicate with all parts of your body. Information is transmitted from neuron to neuron by chemical messengers. Neurons receive information from other neurons through their receptors. Neural receptors are like a TV antenna, but while a TV antenna will pick up any TV signal, neural receptors are very selective. They only recognize particular messages, and ignore all the rest. Morphine was 1,000 times stronger in the brain than in any other part of the body. Could there be special "morphine receptors" on brain neurons?

## THE DISCOVERY OF "MORPHINE RECEPTORS"

In 1972 Dr. Candace Pert and Dr. Solomon Snyder at the Johns Hopkins University School of Medicine were investigating the way in which drugs interacted with brain tissue. One of the problems they were examining was the morphine mystery: How do very small amounts of morphine exert such powerful effects in human beings? The answer seemed obvious to Dr. Pert: There must be nerve cell receptors specifically sensitive to morphine.

An important concept they worked with was the notion of the lock-and-key type bond. The idea, widely accepted by pharmacologists, holds that drugs or hormones cannot interact with a nerve cell until they form a lock-and-key bond with a neural receptor. In other words, the drug or hormone is the "key" that "unlocks" specific actions of the neuron ("lock").

To find out whether there were "morphine receptors" in the

brain, Drs. Pert and Snyder incubated homogenized samples of brain tissue from various regions of the brain with a drug called naloxone.

Naloxone is an "opiate blocker." Although not an opiate-type drug, it "graps at" and tightly bonds to opiate receptors. This prevents opiate drugs (such as morphine) from forming the lock-and-key bond with the receptors. They can't—the naloxone is in the way. Many times patients have been brought to me in hospital emergency rooms in a coma. If I suspected the coma was due to a narcotic overdose, I'd give Narcan (the tradename for naloxone) intravenously. If the coma had in fact been caused by a narcotic overdose, the patient would wake up immediately as the Narcan rapidly "shut out" the narcotic.

But Pert and Snyder were not trying to "shut out" opiates. They wanted to see if the naloxone would bind to anything in the brain tissue; that is, if there were opiate receptors for the nalox-one to "hold onto." If the naloxone was easily washed out of the brain tissue after incubating, it would be assumed there were no receptors for naloxone to bind to.

But the naloxone held on very tightly. There were some type of opiate receptors in the brain! Pert and Snyder found neural receptors no one had ever seen. As Dr. Pert said: "I tried and tried and tried and gotten [sic] nothing and then one day—there they were. I was suddenly looking at something in the brain nobody had ever really known was there before."[1]

Pert and Snyder's 1972 discovery of "morphine receptors" in the brain[2] electrified researchers worldwide. It was later re-ported that high densities of opiate receptors were found in areas of the spinal cord involved in modulating pain.[3] As studies continued at major universities in many countries, it was learned that the opiate receptors are strategically placed in key areas of the brain and spinal cord where they can do the most to relieve pain.

Another interesting finding was that there are lots of opiate receptors in a brain region known as the "limbic system," a collection of brain structures that have long been believed to regulate emotional states. The existance of many opiate receptors in the limbic system may account for the euphoric feeling experi-enced by those who take morphine.

## BUT WHY MORPHINE RECEPTORS?

Why should humans have evolved highly specialized neural receptors for a substance that is not a part of human chemistry? After all, morphine is an alkaloid derived from opium plants—it's not supposed to be in the human brain! Did nature intend for us to become narcotic users? Brain scientists did not think so. But why did morphine receptors exist, and exist in such numbers in strategic areas of the nervous system? Well, if there was a "morphine lock" in the brain, there had to be a "morphine key." The human brain must manufacture a substance very similar to morphine to fit into the opiate receptors. Humans must manufacture some kind of natural opiate.

## THE RACE WAS ON

Scientists did not know exactly what they were looking for, but they raced ahead in one of the most intense searches for a brain chemical in the history of science. A new rush of discoveries began in 1975 with a series of research reports[4] from the University of Aberdeen in Scotland. In that year, Dr. John Hughes and Dr. Hans Kosterlitz found the first of the endorphins! As they stated in their report appearing in the prestigious journal *Brain Research:*

> The morphine-like substance was unevenly distributed in the brain . . . It is suggested that the compound isolated in this investigation forms part of a central pain suppression system . . ."

Hughes and Kosterlitz later learned that they had actually found not one but two morphine-like substances. The chemicals were named methionine-enkephalin and leucine-enkephalin. (Enkephalin is Greek for "in the head.") Each of the enkephalins was a chain of five amino acids, each identical to the other except for one amino acid. Methionine-enkephalin had the amino acid methionine where luecine-enkephalin had the amino acid leucine.

Although Hughes and Kosterlitz are often credited as being the first to discover an endorphin, the nearly simultaneous nature of the rush of the discoveries clouds the issue. In rapid succession researchers announced the discovery of several more substances displaying opiate-like action, including beta-endorphin, alpha-endorphin, dynorphin, and others.

It turns out that scientists had some endorphins sitting on the shelf since 1964, but did not know it. In that year, Choh Hao Li, of the Hormone Research Laboratory at the University of California, San Francisco, and his colleagues found a protein they called beta-lipotropin. No one knew exactly what beta-lipotropin did, so it sat on the shelf until the end of 1975, when Hughes and Kosterlitz announced that methionine-enkephalin was a part of

## AMINO ACID SEQUENCE OF BETA-LIPOTROPIN

H–GLU–LEU–THR–GLY–GLN–ARG–LEU–ARG–GLN–GLY–  10

ASP–GLY–PRO–ASN–ALA–GLY–ALA–ASN–ASP–GLY–  20

GLU–GLY–PRO–ASN–ALA–LEU–GLU–HIS–SER–LEU–  30

LEU–ALA–ASP–LEU–VAL–ALA–ALA–GLU–LYS–LYS–  40

ASP–GLU–GLY–PRO–TYR–ARG–MET–GLU–HIS–PHE–  50

ARG–TRP–GLY–SER–PRO–PRO–LYS–ASP–LYS–ARG–  60

TYR–GLY–GLY–PHE–MET–THR–SER–GLU–LYS–SER–  70

GLN–THR–PRO–LEU–VAL–THR–LEU–PHE–LYS–ASN–  80

ALA–ILE–ILE–LYS–ASN–ALA–TYR–LYS–LYS–GLY–  90

GLU–OH

TYR–GLY–GLY–PHE–MET–

61–65 Met–Enkephalin

TYR–GLY–GLY–PHE–MET–THR–SER–GLU–LYS–SER–

GLN–THR–PRO–LEU–VAL–THR–LEU–PHE–LYS–ASN–

ALA–ILE–ILE–LYS–ASN–ALA–TYR–LYS–LYS–GLY–

GLU

61–91 β-Endorphin

KEY

| | | | | | |
|---|---|---|---|---|---|
| Ala | = Alanine | Ile | = Isoleucine | Ser | = Serine |
| Arg | = Arginine | His | = Histidine | Thr | = Threonine |
| Asn | = Asparagine | Leu | = Leucine | Trp | = Tryptophan |
| Asp | = Aspartic Acid | Lys | = Lysine | Tyr | = Tyrosine |
| Gln | = Glutamine | Met | = Methionine | Val | = Valine |
| Glu | = Glutamic Acid | Phe | = Phenylalanine | | |
| Gly | = Glycine | Pro | = Proline | | |

beta-lipotropin! It seems that beta-lipotropin, which is composed of 91 amino acids, is a precursor, or "parent" of some endorphins. Cells in the nervous system contain different enzymes that "process," or "cut" beta-lipotropin into smaller, neurally active endorphins. When the enzymes "snip off" amino acids number 61 to 91, you get beta-endorphin. Separating amino acids number 61 to 76 produces alpha-endorphin, while cutting out amino acids number 61 to 65 yields methionine-enkephalin.

The entire group of opiate-like substances is referred to as the endorphins. The two enkephalins are sometimes called "small endorphins" because they are, well, they're small compared to the other endorphins.

There are many other substances in the nervous system which may prove to have opiate-like activity. In the coming years we may identify as many as 20 different endorphins.

## LOCK-AND-KEY

The diagram below shows the structural relationship between morphine and endorphins (stylized for presentation). Imagine that the receptor is the "lock" and the chemical messenger is the "key." The morphine key (M) is a pretty close fit; not perfect,

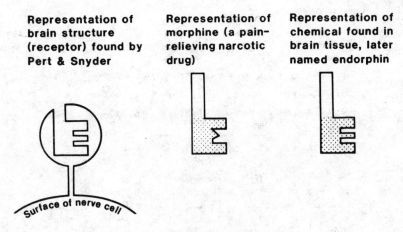

Lock and Key Concept of Neural Receptors

but good enough to "unlock" the receptor and trigger a pain-killing message. But the endorphin "key" (E) is a perfect fit. It opens the "lock" wide open to initiate a powerful antipain message.

Morphine kills pain, there are morphine receptors in the brain and spinal cord, and the endorphins are similar to morphine. Does it all add up? Are the endorphins part of a natural built-in pain-control system? And if they are, why are so many millions of Americans suffering from so much pain?

Well, the best way to find out if endorphins are natural pain killers is to put them to the test. Before we look at the studies, however, let me say a few words about two different kinds of pain.

## GOOD AND BAD PAIN

All pain is bad in the sense that it is unpleasant. But we could not survive for long without the type of pain called acute pain.

Acute pain is part of a vital feedback system. It's your body's way of telling you something is wrong, tissue is being damaged. Acute pain is that sharp, intense pain you feel when you feel when you hit your head, drop something on your foot, or get your hand caught in a closing car door. Acute pain arrives forcefully to grab your attention, tells you something is wrong so you had better do something about it, then gradually leaves. Without acute pain you may not know your body is being damaged. In that sense acute pain is "good pain."

Chronic pain, the "bad pain," does not serve the same useful purpose. Chronic pain can linger for days, months, often years. In most cases, there is no apparent physical reason for the pain. Whereas acute pain is the bearer of bad news, chronic pain is in itself the bad news.

Assaulted by a terrible pain they cannot understand, chronic pain patients often feel helpless and hopeless. They neither eat nor sleep well. Losing faith in medicine, and often in life itself, they may become angry, bitter, and depressed. Pain captures them, body, mind, and soul, thrusting itself into every aspect of their life. Chronic pain often *becomes* their life.

You need acute pain. Chronic pain can ruin you.

## EARLY ENDORPHIN STUDIES DISAPPOINTING

The early studies showed that the enkephalins, especially methionine-enkephalin, killed pain when injected directly into the central nervous system. But there was a problem: The pain relief lasted only 20 minutes or less. Later studies[5] showed there were enzymes in the body that quickly broke the enkephalins up. Apparently, the injected enkephalins were (largely) destroyed by these enzymes within 20 minutes or less. (It was shown that chemically modified enkephalins would resist enzymatic destruction.[6] These artificial enkephalins were hundreds of times stronger than morphine and could be made to last much longer than 20 minutes.)

Other tests showed that beta-endorphin injected into the veins produced a long-lasting analgesia three times stronger than morphine analgesia.[7] And when injected directly into the brain, beta-endorphin was *18 to 50 times stronger than morphine!*[8] Using a sophisticated technique for assessing opiate potency, researchers at Stanford University showed that dynorphin is 50 times more potent than beta-endorphin![9]

These findings were amazing! The endorphins were many, many times more powerful than morphine, the strongest painkiller available! Theoretically the endorphins seemed to be the ultimate answer to chronic pain. Unfortunately, there were several obstacles to be overcome:

1. Endorphin analgesia does not usually last long because the endorphins are continually destroyed by enzymes.
2. To be most effective, endorphins must be injected directly into the brain or spinal cord. This requires complicated, expensive, and dangerous procedures.
3. You could make endorphin "pills" to be swallowed, but the digestive juices in the stomach and gastrointestinal tract would break the endorphins down into individual amino acids (or small chains), that are useless for killing pain.

What about synthetic endorphins? Is it possible to alter endorphins in the laboratory so they can get past the digestive juices and resist endorphin-destroying enzymes? That can be done, but changing even one little part of a chemical can dramatically alter the way it is utilized in the body, the way it interacts with neurons and other body chemicals. A team of European researchers funded by Sandoz Laboratories administered an altered enkephalin called "FK 33-824" to 40 healthy male volunteers. Doses ranged between .10 and 1.2 milligrams. *Every one of the men* experienced a feeling of heaviness in all the muscles of his body, often in conjunction with an oppressive feeling in the chest or a tightening in the throat. A little over half the men experienced flushing of the face or other problems.

Artificial endorphins can solve some problems, but only at the cost of exposing the body and brain to unnatural, potentially dangerous substances.

Despite the problems, scientists continued to delve into the endorphin phenomenon. Let's take a look at some of the endorphin/pain studies.

## THE FIRST STUDIES WITH HUMAN PAIN PATIENTS

A research team at the University of California, Los Angeles, Department of Medicine headed by Dr. Don Catlin, a well-known hormone specialist, was the first to inject endorphins into human pain patients.[10] Three patients suffering from very severe chronic cancer pain were given very small doses of beta-endorphins (one half to several milligrams); much less than a typical dose of aspirin. The patients rated their pain before and after the endorphins. They were also evaluated by a trained observer. Here are the results:

**PATIENT #1**

*Complaint:* Severe chronic pain due to cancer.

*Result:* Complete pain relief within 45 minutes.

*Comments:* No further medication was required for 18 hours.

**PATIENT #2**

*Complaint:* Severe chronic pain due to cancer.

*Result:* Slight reduction in pain.

*Comments:* The observer judged the patient to have experienced good relief within 30 minutes based on the fact that the patient was "talkative and moved more freely than usual."

**PATIENT #3**

*Complaint:* Severe chronic pain due to cancer.

*Result:* Nearly total pain relief within 15 minutes.

*Comments:* The patient's family and physicians reported an "improvement in the patient's mood, as manifested by smiling, loquaciousness, and a less vigilant attitude."

How about side effects? *None of the patients* experienced euphoria, altered sensory perceptions, hallucinations, or other subjective effects associated with morphine and other opiate painkillers. Nor were there any changes in blood pressure, pulse, temperature, respiratory rate, or any abnormal movements or reflex changes. The researchers wrote:

The subjects have been followed for a total of 110 patient days. There have been no adverse reactions that could be attributed to beta-endorphin.

In this study the endorphin was injected into the patient's veins, not into their brains. It is felt that endorphins cannot cross from the blood into the brain, so these encouraging results suggested that beta-endorphin blocked pain by acting on structures or processes outside the brain. If endorphins were this effective when injected into the veins, scientists thought, what would happen if they were delivered directly into the brain?

## ENDORPHINS TO THE BRAIN

In 1978, Drs. Hosobuchi and Li conducted a study in the Department of Neurological Surgery at the University of California, San Francisco.[11] This time beta-endorphin was injected directly into the patient's brains!

The participants were three "hard-core" patients with long-standing excruciating pain. They had already had surgery performed that made possible direct electrical stimulation of certain parts of the brain in an attempt to quell their pain.

### 3 CHRONIC PAIN PATIENTS

*Dosage:*     .20 milligrams (a very small amount)
*Results:*     "A clear analgesic effect was observed" in the participants.
*Comments:*   "Patients were relatively free of pain for four to six hours."
*Side Effects:* None

The dosage level was doubled:

*Dosage:*     .40 milligrams
*Results:*     Pain relief was described as "profound and prolonged."
*Side Effects:* None

These results were nothing short of amazing, especially considering the tiny amounts of beta-endorphins used (less than $1/100$th the standard dose of aspirin). And this without any side effects. There were absolutely no disturbances of vital signs, neurological functions, or behavior in any of the three patients. To the contrary, "they appeared to be more relaxed, cheerful and generally more talkative." There was no evidence of the euphoria associated with morphine and opiate drugs.

## "IT IS REMARKABLE. . . ."

Now let's look at a large study conducted by teams of researchers from the Hiroasko University School of Medicine in Japan and the prestigious Salk Institute in California, including Dr. Roger Guillemin, winner of the Nobel prize and an authority in endorphin chemistry.[12] (As a moderator at the Second International Symposium on the Management of Stress, held in Monte Carlo in 1979, I shared the podium with this distinguished medical researcher.)

The power of beta-endorphin was pitted against some of the most agonizing pain humans can suffer; cancer pain and labor pain accompanying childbirth. This time the endorphin was given intrathecally, which means injected directly into the spinal fluid. Here are the results:

### 14 CANCER PATIENTS

These 14 people had chronic pain that resisted even the most powerful narcotic drugs. The pain was so bad they could not sleep well.

*Dosage:* 3 milligrams

*Results:* All of the patients reported "profound and longlasting complete relief of pain."

*Comments:* It took only five minutes for the analgesia to appear—and it lasted for an average of 33 hours.

*Side Effects:* There were no disturbances in a host of physiologic variables, including respiration, arterial blood-gas changes, nausea, hypotension, hypothermia, catatonia, or muscle rigidity. No abnormalities in the EKG or EEG (heart and brain measurements) were noted.

There were some reports of mild side effects such as passing drowsiness, and "several patients became euphoric."

The results were tremendous. The pain was blocked so rapidly it suggested that beta-endorphin acted directly on opiate receptors in the spinal cord itself, stopping the "pain message" before it ascended to the brain. (Remember, in this study the endorphins were injected into the spinal fluid.)

The second part of the study involved 14 women who were going to have babies by vaginal (normal) delivery. Beta-endorphin was injected directly into the spinal fluid when cervical dilation was, on the average, 6.3 centimeters.

### 14 OBSTETRIC PATIENTS

*Dosage:* 1 milligram

*Results:* 3½ minutes after beta-endorphin was injected, "labor pains in all patients disappeared completely."

*Comments:* Pain relief lasted 12 to 32 hours.

*Side Effects:* No serious side effects—for mother or baby—

were noted. Several women felt mild drowsiness.

## HOW DO ENDORPHINS BLOCK PAIN?

As I mentioned earlier, "pain information" is passed along by neurons in the nervous system. If you were to examine nerve tissue in the brain or spinal cord with a powerful microscope, you would see how nerve cells containing endorphins are positioned to block pain.

Look at the top half of the diagram below. A "pain message" (nerve impulse) is being carried along the pain-sensitive nerve

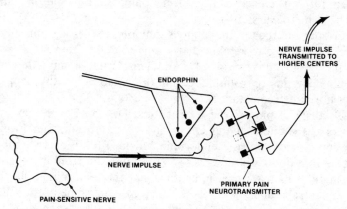

PAIN IMPULSE CAUSES RELEASE OF PRIMARY NEUROTRANSMITTER—PAIN MESSAGE PASSED ON.

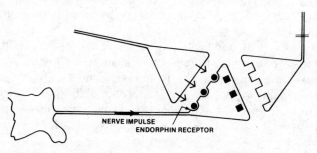

ENDORPHINS BLOCK RELEASE OF PRIMARY NEUROTRANSMITTER—PAIN MESSAGE BLOCKED.

cell. When the "pain message" reaches the end of the nerve cell, pain neurotransmitters (squares) are released. The neurotransmitters bind to their receptor sites in the next nerve cell, and the "pain message" continues on.

Now look at the bottom half of the diagram. This time endorphins (round) are released by an adjacent nerve cell. The endorphins bind to their receptors in the pain-sensitive nerve cell. By locking onto their receptors, the endorphins prevent the pain neurotransmitters (squares) from moving forward. The pain message is blocked.

## IS CHRONIC PAIN CAUSED BY AN ENDORPHIN DEFICIENCY?

Endorphins clearly block chronic pain. But how did the pain get there in the first place? In some cases, such as injury or cancer, the source of the pain is obvious. Still, millions and millions of people have pain that seems to come from nowhere. Are the endorphins involved? And what role, if any, do endorphins play in controlling the pain threshold in healthy people under normal circumstances?

To answer some of these questions, Dr. Jon Levine[13] and a team of researchers at the University of California, San Francisco gave naloxone (the endorphin blocker) to 26 oral surgery patients in a double-blind cross-over study. Naloxone increased the patients' pain ratings, indicating that the endorphins play a role in naturally and spontaneously suppressing some of the pain of dental surgery. Other studies with naloxone, such as one conducted at the National Institute of Health by Dr. Monte Bushsbaum[14] support the idea that endorphins "set the tone" for pain sensitivity.

The studies seem to indicate that the more endorphin activity you have in certain areas of the nervous system, the higher your normal pain threshold will be. Conversely, people with less tolerance for pain might have less endorphin activity in critical areas of the nervous system. Does this mean that those with chronic pain might suffer as they do because of a lack of endorphin activity?

In testing the relationship between chronic pain and endorphins, Drs. Lars Terenius and Agenta Wahlstrom in Sweden[15] found that the activity of a natural "morphine-like factor" was about 50 percent lower in chronic pain patients than in other patients.

Another team of researchers[16] looked for endorphin activity in spinal fluid samples taken from 80 chronic pain patients. Here's what they found:

1. Chronic pain patients had lower endorphin levels than did normal, healthy volunteers.
2. When the pain patients were grouped according to whether their pain was of "mental origin" or "organic" origin (traceable to a physical problem), those with organic pain syndromes had lower endorphin levels.
3. The patients who had lower pain thresholds and less tolerance to pain also had relatively less endorphin activity.

In another study[17] conducted along these lines, both the beta-endorphin and beta-lipotropin levels in the blood and spinal fluid were sampled in 24 chronic pain patients. (beta-lipotropin, you remember, is the precursor of beta-endorphin.)

When the researchers looked at the blood samples, they found that the pain patients had 87 percent less beta-endorphin than the pain-free subjects did, and just over two thirds less beta-lipotropin. In the spinal fluid, pain patients had half the beta-endorphin pain-free participants did, while beta-lipotropin levels were similar for both groups.

These researchers suggested that the pain patients' endorphin levels may be abnormally low because of uncontrolled oversecretion. In other words, the "recurrent stimulus" of "chronic pain" may be causing them to "use up" their endorphins. It's also possible that overactive endorphin-destroying enzymes are responsible for the shortfall.

The endorphin–chronic pain connection was also examined in a study of migraine headaches.[18] Endorphin levels were measured in normal subjects, in people with common migraines, and in those with an advanced form of migraine. Compared to the control (healthy) group, endorphin levels in the common migraine group were 50 percent lower, and 80 percent lower in the advanced migraine group (as measured in the cerebrospinal fluid). In other words, the worse the migraine condition, the lower the endorphin level.

Dr. Ivy Fettes of the University of Toronto has looked at the relationship between endorphins and migraine headaches in his not-yet-published study involving 11 "classical" migraine sufferers, 22 with common migraine, and 29 healthy controls. Those with classical migraines had an average of only one-third the beta-endorphin found in the blood of the others. Other migraine-endorphin studies[19] have found a similar relationship between migraine pain and endorphins.

Is it possible that low endorphin levels may contribute to arthritis? This interesting hypothesis is supported by research conducted at Case Western Reserve University by Dr. Charles Denko, recently published in the *Journal of Rheumatology*.[20] Blood samples were drawn from patients with a wide variety of arthritic conditions. Endorphin levels were low in patients with osteoarthritis, rheumatoid arthritis, gout, systemic lupus erythematosus, ankylosing spondylitis, and psoratic arthritis.

Dr. Denko suggested that the endorphins are part of man's protective mechanisms for fighting inflammatory arthritis. If this is indeed the case, a low level of endorphins may make it harder for a person to resist arthritic inflammation. We need a lot more study in this area, but it appears that some of the following factors may contribute to arthritic pain and inflammation:

1. decreased activity of endorphins/enkephalins in the bone joints (synovial fluid);
2. extra-active endorphin-destroying enzymes in joints; and/or
3. a deficiency of endorphin precursors in the pituitary and/or adrenal glands.

In light of these possibilities, the use of DLPA to treat arthritis may constitute a "biologically appropriate" therapy. By that I mean that unlike arthritis drugs, DLPA might actually get to the "root" of the problem; lack of sufficiently high levels of endorphins.

The various studies suggest a strong link between chronic pain and an endorphin deficiency. More research is needed, but it is reasonable to suspect that if endorphin levels in the nervous system fall below a certain critical level, a person will experience pain. And the pain will be felt despite the absence of a disease or injury to prompt the pain.

## STRESS, INJURY, AND ENDORPHINS

The endorphins are marvelous natural pain-killers, but where are they when you accidentally smash your hand with a hammer? The endorphins do not block acute pain of this nature, but they apparently set the pain perception threshold on a constant, or "tonic," basis. (Sudden acute injury, such as automobile accidents or battle wounds, can "switch on" the endorphin system to block pain, but the surge in endorphin activity subsides within a short period of time and pain begins.)

An interesting aspect of the endorphin story is what is called the "autoanalgesia" phenomenon, or self-regulated pain reduction. Autoanalgesia refers to an increase in the pain threshold that occurs with repeated exposure to painful and stressful events of an acute, not chronic, nature. If you subject laboratory animals to a painful stimulus, such as electric shock, over and over, their pain threshold rises—they can withstand more pain than previously was the case. Solid evidence suggests this happens because acute stress (electrical shock) activates endorphins. Their endorphins being more active, the animals can tolerate more pain. Naloxone, the endorphin blocker, can prevent and or reverse autoanalgesia. This suggests that a person's ability to cope with stress may depend on his or her endorphin levels. Without sufficient endorphins an individual may be more vulnerable to the ravages of stress. If this is the case, building up your endorphin levels may help protect you against stress. (In chapter 14 I will discuss using the power of the mind to increase your endorphins for protection against stress.)

## CONCLUSION

There you have the endorphin story, in a nutshell. The discovery of the endorphin hormones has unquestionably been one of the most important breakthroughs in modern science. Their discovery has prompted a whole constellation of related findings which have greatly expanded our knowledge of how the nervous system works. Assisted and protected by DLPA, the endorphins are opening a new and very pleasant chapter in the long and often frustrating history of pain relief. Now let's look at DLPA, the endorphin "shield."

# 12

## DLPA: BRAIN-ACTIVE NUTRIENT

In some respects, it seemed as if the endorphins were destined to become one of the biggest "almosts" in the history of pain relief. Although much more powerful than our strongest analgesics, they were impractical and costly to deal with, difficult and dangerous to deliver to the appropriate parts of the body. No, endorphins did not seem to be the answer. It seemed as if we had no choice but to accept chronic pain as part of our lives, at least for the present.

That changed in 1978. Dr. Seymour Ehrenpreis[1] and a team of researchers at the Chicago Medical School tried a new approach. Instead of giving pain patients more endorphins, why not try to protect the endorphins they already had? Was there a way to slow down the "endorphin-chewing" enzymes in the body, a method of giving extra "life" to the endorphins?

Earlier researchers had found that DPA (and, to a slight degree, LPA as well) inhibits an enzyme called carboxypeptidase A, one of the "endorphin-chewers." Ehrenpreis reasoned that DPA might block pain by inhibiting this endorphin-destroying enzyme. He was right.

Hundreds of mice were injected with DPA over a 9-day period. Then Ehrenpreis measured whether or not pain was blocked by clocking the amount of time the mice would remain on a hot surface.

DPA blocked pain in 70 percent of the mice, and moreover, the analgesic effects became stronger with time! The DPA was blocking more pain on the ninth day than it did on the first day. That's the opposite of what happens with conventional painkillers. The tolerance that develops with the use of narcotic drugs did not occur with DPA.

Furthermore, none of the mice experienced side effects, which is quite surprising considering that every pain-killer and antidepressant drug we know of, even aspirin, has some, sometimes many, side effects. And finally, DPA seemed to be able to work with, to heighten, the effects of other medications.

## DLPA FOR HUMAN PAIN PATIENTS

Dr. Ehrenpreis and his team were so encouraged by the results with laboratory animals they decided to test DPA on human pain patients. They chose 10 chronic pain patients, people who had experienced little or no relief with conventional pain

### ANALGESIA IN HUMAN PAIN PATIENTS IN RESPONSE TO D-PHENYLALANINE

| Condition | Took DLPA For | Result | Prior Treatment |
|---|---|---|---|
| Low back pain for several years | 3 days | Good relief | Spinal fusion, percutaneous nerve stimulation |
| Low back pain for several years | 3 days | Good to excellent relief | Surgery, percutaneous nerve stimulation |
| Low back pain for several years | 3 days | Excellent relief | Conventional pain drugs |
| Low back and neck pain for several years | 3 days | Complete relief | Acupuncture |
| Cervical osteoarthritis and post-operative pain | 2 days | Good relief | |
| Osteoarthritis for five years | Maintained | Excellent relief | Conventional pain drugs |
| Rheumatoid arthritis for several years | 7 days | Considerable relief | Conventional pain drugs |
| Migraine headaches for several years | 2 days | Good relief | |
| Whiplash pain for two years | 3 days | Complete relief for one month | Conventional pain drugs |
| Fibrositis of muscle | 3 days | Complete relief for two days | Conventional pain drugs |

Adapted from *Advances in Pain Research and Therapy,* Vol. 3, eds. J. J. Bonica, J. C. Liebeskind, and D. G. Albe-Fessard, New York, Raven Press, 1978, pp. 479–88.

therapies. The results of this first study on humans were published in 1978 in the prestigious pain research journal, *Advances in Pain Research and Therapy*. What were the results? "Good to excellent relief of pain was noted in every case."

Phenylalanine relieved long-standing chronic pain without adverse side effects, without addiction, without the development of tolerance, and without interfering with the patients' life styles! We doctors have nothing in our black bags that can produce comparable results.

This first study on human pain patients was not the last. Dr. Ehrenpreis and his collaborators replicated and extended the preliminary findings.[2] From France, in 1981, came the report of a study testing the effectiveness of D-phenylalanine in chronic pain patients.[3] (Included in this study were cancer patients.) The analgesia was so complete and long lasting that they could discontinue other pain treatments and even stop taking the DPA for 10 days at a time. No side effects were noted. In 1983 Dr. Reuben Balagot[4], a neurosurgeon at the Chicago Veterans Administration Hospital, reported on a DPA/pain study involving 43 patients. These were people suffering the "chronic pain" of osteoarthritis, rheumatoid arthritis, headaches, or other disorders. DPA "provided good relief in chronic pain patients. . . ." These and other studies leave no doubt that DPA is a powerful analgesic.

## PROTECTING ENDORPHINS WITH DLPA

The initial research raised some new questions: Which enzyme, or group of enzymes, was actually degrading endorphins? Were all endorphins attacked by the same enzyme(s)? Where exactly did DPA fit into the picture?

To answer some of these questions, Dr. Ehrenpreis[5] and his team took tissue samples from four regions of the nervous system and incubated them with either beta-endorphin or methionine-enkephalin. They measured how long it took for enzymes in the tissue samples to chew up these two endorphins. Then they ran the test again, this time adding DPA in the tissue samples along with one of the endorphins. It took *longer* for the enzymes to take apart the endorphins when DPA was added. The researchers did not care *which or how many* enzymes were breaking up endorphins, or *which or how many* enzymes DPA was slowing down. *All* the enzymes were lumped together as the researchers empirically showed that DPA successfully inhibited the whole group of endorphin-destroyers.

The graph below shows how DPA inhibits the enzyme(s) that destroy beta-endorphin and methionine-enkephalin. DPA really puts the break on the enkephalin-destroying enzyme(s).

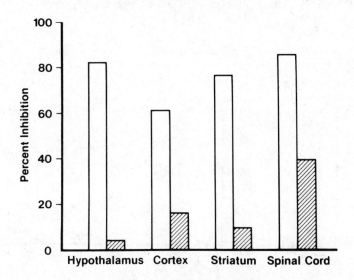

**Inhibition of Enkephalin-Destroying☐ and β-Endorphin-Destroying▨ Enzymes in Nervous System Tissue**

**Graph shows how much two types of endorphin-destroying enzymes are slowed down or inhibited by D-phenylalanine**

Adapted from: Ehrenpreis, S., Greenberg, J., Kubota, K., and Myles, S. Analgesic properties of D-phenylalanine, bacitracin, and puromycin in mice: Relationship to inhibition of enkephalinase and beta-endorphinase. In: Advances in Endogenous and Exogenous Opioids: Proceedings of the International Narcotic Research Conference. Kodancha, Tokyo, pp 279-281, 1981

(The hypothalamus, cortex, striatum, and spinal cord are all regions of the nervous system.)

## INCREASING ENDORPHINS WITH DLPA

Knowing that DPA protected endorphins, the next step was to see if it would actually *increase* endorphin levels. To test this, Dr. Balagot[6] injected several groups of mice with DPA. A control group received no DPA.

One group of mice was sacrificed 90 minutes later, and the levels of methionine-enkephalin in three regions of the central nervous system (periaqueductal gray, cerebral cortex, and spinal cord) were measured. Another group of mice was sacrificed and measured on the second day, and a third group on the sixth day. As you can see below, the levels of methionine-enkephalin in the periaqueductal gray just about tripled within 90 minutes following the DPA injection, and remained about twice as high six days later!

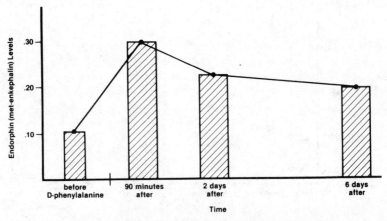

Adapted from: Balagot, R., Ehrenpreis, S., Kubota, K., and Greenberg, J. Analgesia in mice and humans by D-phenylalanine: Relation to inhibition of enkephalin degredation and enkaphalin levels. In: Advances in Pain Research and Therapy, Vol. 5. Edited by J. J. Bonica et al. Ravon. New York. pp 289-293. 1983.

This study demonstrated that DPA has extremely long-lasting effects on at least one endorphin in a critical region of the brain. This very persistent biochemical effect may explain why DLPA reduces pain for weeks at a time *after* its use has been discontinued.

## HOW DOES DLPA WORK?

### Hypothetical Convergence of Factors Contributing to Analgesic Actions of DLPA

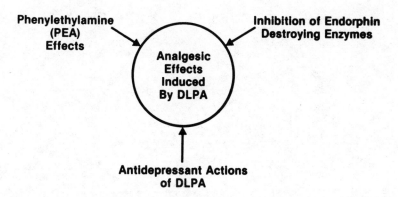

Present biochemical evidence suggests that DLPA works to kill pain in several ways:

1. **Enzyme inhibition:** DLPA extends the life of your endorphins by slowing up the endorphin-chewing enzymes.
2. **Phenylethylamine (PEA) Effects:** PEA is a chemical produced in the brain that can sensitize endorphin receptors to endorphins. That is, PEA can make it easier for endorphins and their receptors to form the necessary lock-and-key bond. In that way PEA makes the endorphins already present in certain areas more effective. There is also evidence that PEA can trigger the release of endorphins on its own. As you'll see on page 173, PEA is a breakdown product of phenylalamine.
3. **Antidepressant Effects:** Pain is worsened by depression. DLPA helps by relieving depression through PEA, one of its breakdown products. This, in turn, helps "lighten" the pain.

DLPA may block pain by acting at two levels of the central nervous system. Dr. Ehrenpreis's and Dr. Balagot's work suggests that DLPA may increase the activity of methionine-enkephalin in the periaqueductal gray, and of beta-endorphin and methionine-enkephalin in the spinal cord. It seems that DLPA inhibits the endorphinase ("endorphin-chewers") and enkephalinase ("enkephalin-chewers") in these regions, giving extra "life" to the endorphins present. Thus, DLPA may assist the endorphins in blocking pain in both the brain stem and the spinal cord.

## THE DUAL ACTION OF DLPA IN ANALGESIA

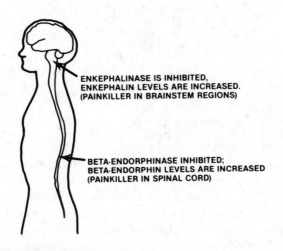

ENKEPHALINASE IS INHIBITED,
ENKEPHALIN LEVELS ARE INCREASED.
(PAINKILLER IN BRAINSTEM REGIONS)

BETA-ENDORPHINASE INHIBITED;
BETA-ENDORPHIN LEVELS ARE INCREASED
(PAINKILLER IN SPINAL CORD)

## PLACEBO OR DLPA?

A placebo is a sugar pill, something that is not really medicine. But the power of the mind is such that if people believe something, like a placebo, is going to help them, as many as 30 to 40 percent of them will get better. Was the placebo effect responsible for the amazing results seen, for example, in Dr. Ehrenpreis's study on human pain patients? Several facts argue against this:

1.  All of the patients had tried various pain pills and/or therapies. If they were susceptible to the placebo effects, they would have responded with this effect to the other treatments.

2. The placebo effect is generally effective in only 30 to 40 percent of patients. *All* the patients responded in Dr. Ehrenpreis's study.
3. The placebo effect occurs very quickly, usually within several hours. But it took *at least* two days for pain relief to develop in these patients.

D-phenylalanine was put to a specific placebo test by Dr. Keith Budd[7], an anaesthesiologist in the Department of Anesthetics at the Royal Infirmary in London. Adults with "long standing intractable pain" that was "resistant to previous drug and physical therapy" were enrolled in this double-blind controlled study.

This was not a test of DPA's overall effectiveness. The point was to see which was blocking pain: DPA or the placebo effect. D-phenylalanine proved to be significantly stronger than the placebo.

## PHENYLALANINE

Before closing the book on DLPA, for now, anyway, let's take a look at a few very important items. This key information helps demonstrate that phenylalanine is a safe, nutritional substance the human body is well-equipped to deal with.

### Structure

Earlier I menationed that DLPA is a 50/50 mixture of DPA and LPA. Here is a representation of the two PA forms:

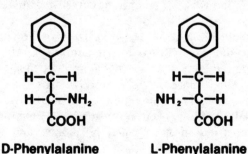

**D-Phenylalanine**        **L-Phenylalanine**

KEY
H = hydrogen     N = nitrogen
C = carbon       O = oxygen

What's the difference? Look for the amine group ($NH_2$). On the D-form it's on the right, while on the L-form it's on the left. The two are mirror images of each other; identical but backwards. You cannot superimpose one upon the other. They're like your right and left hands; the same, but different. This seemingly minor structural difference makes a world of functional difference.

## Absorption

We do not fully understand how the PA you eat is absorbed and transported within your body. Several studies have, however, shown that both D- and L-phenylalanine quickly enter the blood stream. Peak blood levels occur in about 1 hour, then taper off. Although some health professionals have suggested that the presence of LPA may interfere with absorption of the D-form, several studies clearly show that this is not the case, even when the L-form is present in large amounts.[8]

## Metabolism

What happens to phenylalanine once it is inside your body? The diagram below outlines PA's metabolic pathways; that is, the different conversions it may undergo in the body.

As you can see, D-phenylalanine can be converted into L-phenylalanine by way of phenypyruvic acid. This is an essential transformation because the body's cells use the L-, not the D-form to make protein. Thus, DPA can be used for protein synthesis or for therapeutic duties. DPA may also be converted to phenylethylamine (PEA), which is involved in mood regulation and depression.

L-phenylalanine is used to synthesize proteins, to manufacture tyrosine, and can also be converted into PEA. Although DPA can be changed to LPA, the L-form cannot be converted into the D-form. This particular conversion only "works" one way.

Your body is well designed to metabolize DLPA. Most of the DLPA you take orally is used in routine body functions (protein synthesis, construction of enzymes, hormones, and neurotransmitters).

A portion of the D-form in DLPA is converted into the L-form and fed into routine metabolic pathways. Another portion is simply excreted into the urine unchanged. But some of the DPA is

## Metabolism of D-Phenylalanine

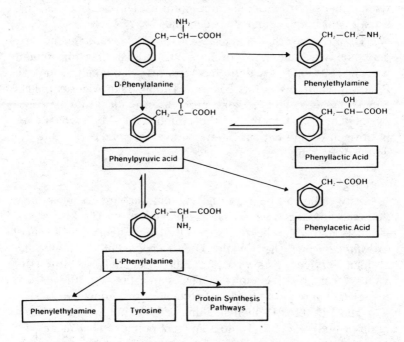

not used in any of these ways. Instead, it goes to protect the endorphins.

For the most part, DPA is "invisible to," that is, does not interact with, just about all of the body's metabolic machinery—except crucial endorphin-destroying enzymes. This is a lucky coincidence for millions of people suffering from chronic pain and depression.

### Requirements

Dr. William Rose of the University of Illinois is one of the world's foremost experts on amino acid metabolism. (Metabolism is the buildup and breakdown of chemical substances in your body, the way chemicals are used to build, maintain, and fuel your body.) He found that adults require, on the average, a *minimum* of 1.1 grams of LPA a day to meet the body's metabolic needs. Most of the PA in our food is in the L-form, so it's not surprising that DPA alone will not satisfy your phenylalanine requirements. DLPA, containing both the D- and L-forms, will satisfy your body's dietary PA demands.

Dr. Rose concluded a series of studies by recommending a daily phenylalanine intake of 2.2 grams, stating that this amount was certainly safe[9]. We don't have to worry about getting enough PA from our foods in this country. The average American meal containing meat and/or dairy products provides anywhere between 0.5 to 2.0 grams of the amino acid. My own studies performed on my patients show an average intake of 3.0 to 5.0 grams of PA daily.

## Toxicity

Any chemical, be it a drug, vitamin, enzyme, or what have you, can be dangerous if you take enough of it. The key is how much is harmful. The *Registery of Toxic Effects of Chemical Substances,* published by the U.S. Department of Health and Human Services, lists what are called Lethal Dose 50 (LD50) values for nearly all chemicals. That's an estimate of the amount of a chemical required to kill 50 percent of the animals tested.

The LD50 for D-phenylalanine is 5,452 milligrams per kilogram of body weight. (1 kilogram = 2.2 pounds) That means if a group of test animals weighed an average of one kilogram each, you would have to inject each of them with 5,452 milligrams of DPA to kill half of them. Extrapolating from these figures, the LD50 for a 154-pound person is roughly 350,000 milligrams, an enormously large figure. It would be very difficult to overdose on DPA.

The LD50 for L-phenylalanine is 5,287 milligrams per kilogram of body weight. Here is a chart comparing the toxicity of DLPA to some common nutritional/dietary supplements:

## WHY DON'T PATIENTS BECOME ADDICTED TO DLPA?

We know that injecting endorphins directly into the brain causes dependence. We also know that DLPA works by increasing the amount of endorphins available. So why don't humans become addicted to DLPA?

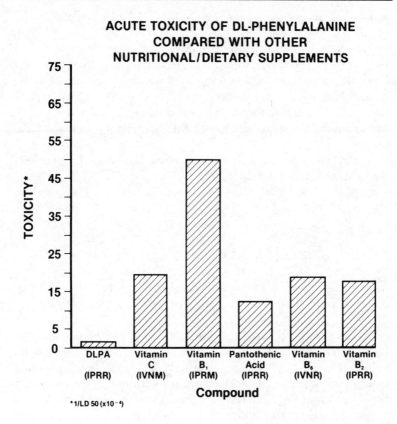

ACUTE TOXICITY OF DL-PHENYLALANINE
COMPARED WITH OTHER
NUTRITIONAL/DIETARY SUPPLEMENTS

*1/LD 50 (x10⁻⁴)

A research team headed by Dr. Yasudo Jacquet of the New York State Research Institute for Neurochemistry[10] set up a bioassay system to measure the opiate-like effects of beta-endorphin (ileum contraction inhibition). They found that opiate-like effects became progressively smaller each time the endorphin was administered—in other words, simulated tolerance developed. Then they added an extract prepared from brain tissue: Tolerance did not develop. Apparently there is something in the brain, a *built-in mechanism,* that prevents acute tolerance to endogenous endorphins (your own endorphins). Nature seems not to have wanted us to become hooked on our own endorphins.

If we have a built-in antitolerance mechanism, how come injecting endorphins into the brain can lead to tolerance? It is likely that the relatively large amounts of endorphins used—up to hundreds of times the amount normally present in the brain—simply overwhelm the protective devices.

Dr. Jeffrey Bland, Research Director of the Linus Pauling Institute, in collaboration with the Palo Alto Veteran's Administration Hospital, is conducting a highly divided dosage experiment. Bland and other scientists feel this dosage schedule will be beneficial for the small fraction of patients who fail to respond to DLPA.

Although I will watch these studies carefully, the previous studies, and more importantly, my experience with patients, suggest the dosage schedule I have worked out is "just what the doctor ordered."

## SPECIAL NOTE ON DLPA DOSAGE

Most of the patients on my DLPA Program take two or three doses of DLPA a day (during the "on" part of the on/off schedule). DLPA does not help a small number of people. Some researchers hypothesize these people fail to respond because the DLPA is cleared from their blood too rapidly to be of therapeutic value. It's felt that putting these patients on a highly divided dosage schedule (*e.g.*, 6 doses a day) will maintain sufficiently high blood levels of DLPA. This approach works well with Parkinson's Disease patients taking L-DOPA.

## CONCLUSION

This chapter barely peeks under the cover of the volumes that could be written on DLPA. I've hardly touched upon the many aspects of this fascinating story. I hope I've given you enough information to pique your curiosity and to convince you that DLPA is a very safe and effective alternative to conventional pain therapies.

# 13

# QUESTIONS AND ANSWERS

### What Is DLPA?

DL-phenylalanine (DLPA) is a special form of an essential amino acid called phenylalanine.

### What Is an "Essential Amino Acid"?

Essential amino acids are amino acids that your body cannot make; you must get them from your diet. There are eight essential amino acids (nine for children).

### What Is an Amino Acid?

Amino acids are the building blocks for your body's protein. They are combined in many different ways to form various proteins and other substances.

### What Is PA?

Phenylalanine (PA) is an amino acid.

### What Is DPA?

D-phenylalanine (DPA) is a form of PA.

### What Is LPA?

L-phenylalanine (LPA) is a form of PA.

### What's the Difference Between PA, DPA, LPA, and DLPA?

They all refer to phenylalanine (PA) which comes in two forms, the "right" and "left" forms. The "right" and "left" forms are essentially mirror images of each other—identical but backwards. DPA is the "right" form and LPA the "left" form. DLPA is a name for a particular formulation of phenylalanine, a 50/50 mixture of DPA and LPA.

### What Does DPA Do?

DPA is the active antichronic pain and antidepression ingredient in DLPA. It provides long-lasting and profound relief from many kinds of chronic pain, arthritis, and depression, as well as from premenstrual syndrome (PMS) and other medical problems.

### What Does LPA Do?

L-phenylalanine is used by your body to make various proteins, enzymes, and other substances you need for good health. (Some researchers also feel LPA has very mild antichronic pain and depression effects.)

### If DPA Is the Active Pain Killing Part, Why Take DLPA? Why Not Just Take DPA?

Phenylalanine's ability to fight pain and depression depend on how much DPA is present. It's true that only 50 percent of DLPA is actually DPA, so you have to take twice as much DLPA to get the same effect. But DPA is 10 times more expensive than DLPA, and it's not produced on a commercial basis. DL-phenylalanine is just as effective as DPA when equivalent amounts of the D-form are given.

### You Said DLPA Is an Amino Acid. Does That Mean I Need It for Good Nutrition?

In order to stay healthy and alive, you must eat enough LPA. There is lots of LPA in food, so we usually don't have to worry about getting enough. DL-phenylalanine is 50 percent LPA, so taking DLPA gives you even more LPA.

### Where Does Phenylanaline Come From?

It comes from the food you eat. Most of the PA in food is LPA. Phenylalanine can also be synthesized in the laboratory.

### How Does DLPA Kill Pain?

DLPA does not kill pain. What DLPA does is protect the endorphins, your body's natural pain-control system.

### Protects Them from What?

There are enzymes in your body that "chew up" your endorphins, making them useless for blocking pain and relieving depression. DLPA slows these enzymes down, giving your endorphins more time to act.

### What Are Endorphins?

The endorphins are morphinelike substances produced by your body. They block pain signals moving through your nervous system. They can also "lift" your mood.

### How Many Endorphins Are There?

We won't know for sure until more studies are completed, but there may be as many as 20 endorphins.

### Is DLPA an Endorphin?

No. DLPA is a nutritional substance. Endorphins are morphinelike chemicals produced in your body.

### What's the Connection Between DLPA and Endorphins?

DLPA, an amino acid, protects the endorphins, your natural, built-in painkillers.

### Are the Endorphins Really Strong Painkillers?

Yes! One of the endorphins, called beta-endorphin, is 18 to 50 times stronger than morphine, the strongest painkiller we have.

### Why Bother with DLPA? Endorphins Are the Real Painkillers, So Why Not Take Endorphin Pills or Something Similar?

That's a good idea, but it doesn't work. You see, endorphins are chains made of amino acids. Amino acid chains are broken into bits (digested) in the stomach and intestines. It takes a whole endorphin "chain" to kill pain; the pieces of the chain won't work separately.

### What About an Endorphin Shot? That Would Take Care of the Problem, Wouldn't It?

Yes, you can bypass the problem of endorphin pills being "broken up' and inactivated by digestive juices by using endorphin injections. But to be really effective, endorphins would have to be injected directly into the brain or spinal cord—that's where the painkilling action takes place. Injections into the brain or spinal cord are difficult, costly, and dangerous.

### Is DLPA Dangerous?

No. DLPA is a nutrient your body is well adapted to handle. DLPA is on the U.S. Government's Generally Regarded As Safe (GRAS) list.

### Is DLPA Habit-Forming?

Not at all. In fact, most people find that they can reduce their dosage, and even stop using it for periods of time.

### Doesn't the Pain Return When You Stop Using It?

DLPA works by increasing the activity of your endorphins. When you stop taking DLPA, your endorphins are still more active. So DLPA continues killing pain even *after* you stop taking it. That's why many of my patients are on an on/off schedule, taking it for a week or 10 days, then not taking it for a couple of weeks.

### Does DLPA Have Side Effects?

A very few people have reported feeling overly "excited" or jittery after taking DLPA. Taking DLPA on a full stomach eliminates this problem.

### Is That Why You Have Your Patients Take DLPA With Meals?

Yes. I tell them to take their DLPA with their meal, or within an hour of finishing the meal.

### Is it a Good Idea to Kill Pain? Don't We Need Some Pain?

DLPA does not block acute pain, the "messenger pain" that warns you some part of your body is being damaged. DLPA works against useless, long-term (chronic) pain.

### Does DLPA Interfere with My Other Medicine?

No. DLPA can normally be combined with other common drugs, therapies, acupuncture, chiropractic, etc. In fact, DLPA often *works with* your other medicine, making it stronger. (Those taking monoamine oxidase inhibitors should not take DLPA—see your physician.)

### How About DLPA and Aspirin?

DLPA and aspirin make a good team. Studies have shown that this combination is very effective in fighting chronic pain and arthritis.

### Does DLPA Also Relieve Depression?

Yes. DLPA increases the levels of your endorphins, of norepinephrine, and of phenylethlyamine, in your body. These natural substances found in your body are your "home made" brain stimulants, mood regulators, and antidepressants. DLPA works by assisting all three of these substances in fighting depression.

### How Effective Is DLPA in the Treatment of Depression?

Many clinical studies have shown DLPA to be 80–90 percent effective in treating depression. Researchers report "excellent" to "complete" relief of symptoms in most cases.

### Is DLPA Like A Stimulant Drug? Is That How It Relieves Depression?

No. DLPA is not a stimulant drug. It relieves depression by assisting natural antidepressants in your nervous system.

### Is DLPA Better Than a Drug?

Many studies have shown DLPA to be as strong as, or stronger than prescription and nonprescription medicines for pain, arthritis, and depression. Not only that, but DLPA does not have the serious side effects seen with the drugs.

### My Doctor Said He Never Heard of DLPA and Didn't Seem to Know Much About Endorphins.

Our scientific knowledge is growing very rapidly. Many physicians, busy treating patients, simply cannot keep up with all the new advances. The DLPA phenomenon is a recent one many doctors are not yet familiar with.

### Is There a Difference in the Way DLPA Affects Men and Women?

No difference has been documented. DLPA seems to work equally well for either sex.

### How About Children? Can I Use DLPA for My Child?

I do not recommend treating children with DLPA simply

because as an internist and cardiologist, I have little experience with children. Furthermore, the effect of DLPA on children has not, to my knowledge, been studied. Although there is no reason to suspect DLPA would harm children, I prefer to wait until the appropriate tests have been conducted.

### Will DLPA Help Me Even If I Don't Give up Junk Food?

Yes. DLPA can relieve chronic pain and depression, even if you do not change your diet. But remember, the state of your general health affects your pain or depression. Dr. Fox's DLPA Program builds up your body and mind while relieving your pain and depression. In some cases I haven't even had to use the DLPA; the rest of my DLPA Program was sufficient. Using DLPA without the rest of my Program is fighting the enemy with one hand tied behind your back.

### How About My Sex Life? Will DLPA Help?

Many depressed patients lose interest in sex. And sex is too difficult or uncomfortable for many pain and arthritis patients. If a lack of interest in, or ability to enjoy sex is due to depression or pain, DLPA can help by relieving the pain or depression.

### I Took DLPA in the Morning and My Back Still Hurt at Night. How Come It Didn't Cure My Back?

DLPA is not fast acting, like aspirin. It takes at least two days, and often as long as several weeks for DLPA to have effect. You have to give it a chance to work.

### I Have Dysmenorrhea. Does DLPA Help?

DLPA relieves the painful uterine cramps known as dysmenorrhea.

### How About for Amenorrhea?

Amenorrhea is a lack of menses. DLPA has no effect on amenorrhea.

### Should I Take DLPA for My Diabetes?

DLPA is not a treatment for diabetes. But I often put my diabetic patients on the other elements of my DLPA Program. The Antistress Diet, Mental Blueprints, and PA Exercise have helped my diabetic patients control their blood sugar, lose weight, and build excellent general health.

### If Someone Gets Hurt, Say, Gets Their Hand Caught in a Car Door, Should They Take DLPA?

DLPA works against chronic pain, not acute pain. The short-term pain you feel when you injure yourself is acute pain.

### What Does DLPA Do For Arthritis?

Two things: DLPA relieves the pain and reduces inflammation and swelling. Arthritics on my DLPA Antiarthritis Plan often regain use of "frozen" joints they have been unable to use for years.

### On/Off Schedule? What Is That?

DLPA is very long acting; its effects last up to three or four weeks after you stop taking it. On/off means you take it until you've felt good for a week, then stop taking it until you need it again. Most of my patients are on DLPA for a week, then off for two or three weeks.

### A Friend Told Me She Took DLPA For Her Back Pain But It Didn't Work.

Nothing is 100 percent effective. When my patients tell me they don't think DLPA is helping, I check to make sure they are taking the dose prescribed for them, taking it at the right time, and are using certified DLPA.

### Certified DLPA? What Is That?

Unfortunately, some individuals or companies are not above selling faulty or phony products. Some of the stuff sold as DLPA has actually been LPA, other amino acids, feed-grade DL-phenylalaline, or otherwise impure. You will not experience the benefits unless you use certified DLPA. Check with your physician or pharmacist to make sure you are getting the real thing.

### Are There Any People Who Should Not Use DLPA?

Yes, pregnant and lactating women should not use DLPA. Neither should anyone with the genetic disease known as phenylketonuria (PKU), or anyone on a phenylalanine-restricted diet.

Persons on a monoamine oxidase inhibitor should not use phenylalanine.

### Do I Have to See a Doctor, or Can I Just Take DLPA?

DLPA is available without a prescription in vitamin and health food stores. If you are considering taking DLPA, I suggest you discuss DLPA and my DLPA Program with your physician.

### My DLPA Is Helping My Pain a Lot. Can I Stop Taking My Other Medicine?

Discuss *all* changes in your medication with your physician. A doctor wants to know what his or her patients are taking—vitamins, drugs, everything.

### Does the L-Phenylalanine in DLPA Interfere with the Anti-pain or Antidepressant Effects of the D-Part of DLPA?

Not at all. Once DLPA dissolves in the stomach, the D- and L-forms go their separate ways in the body.

### I've Had Osteoarthritis for 18 Years and Recently Began Taking DLPA. I Feel Good Now, But I'm Afraid to Stop Taking It Because I'm Afraid the Pain Will Come Back. It Is Really All Right to Just Stop Taking It?

Yes! It may sound strange, but none of my arthritic patients have to take DLPA on a continual basis. Some only need to take DLPA one week out of every month. There is little, if any, chance your pain will return right after you stop taking it.

### I Have a Pain Condition Caused by a Car Accident I Had Several Years Ago. The Pain, in My Back, is Only There One Week before My Menstrual Period—Just Like Clockwork. Since I Know When the Pain Is Going to Start, Should I Take DLPA Right Before?

Good idea. What you're suggesting is a preventive strategy—block the pain before it even starts. I've treated several patients with similar "recurrent" pain problems. When they take DLPA about one week before the pain is due, it never shows up.

### Are Any Medical Doctors Using DLPA for Their Patients?

Yes. Many of my surgical colleagues tell me they give their patients DLPA every day for a week or 10 days prior to surgery.

This reduces the amount of pain the patients feel after the surgery. Some gynecologists have used it to treat PMS, and some psychiatrists are using DLPA in the treatment of depression.

### How Safe Is DLPA?

Very safe. To begin with, the amounts of DL-phenylalanine used as part of the treatment for chronic pain, depression, arthritis, and premenstrual syndrome (PMS) are well within the range of daily amino acid requirements recommended by Dr. William C. Rose, the world's foremost expert on amino acid requirements. For example, the amount of L-phenylalanine taken on the DLPA Program is about equal to the amount you get from eating a peanut butter sandwich. And because the DLPA is taken in smaller, divided doses with all the other amino acids in your meals, it will not cause an amino acid imbalance in your diet. In fact, it will serve a nutritive purpose.

The DL- form of phenylalanine is an extraordinarily nontoxic food substance. The scientific studies and clinical experience with DLPA indicate it is very safe. Among the many patients I have treated with DLPA, only one has complained of any ill-effects (nervousness). And don't forget that most patients are on an on/off schedule with DLPA, only taking it one out of every two to four weeks. That means your average daily dose is very low—that increases the margin of safety.

But is anything absolutely safe 100 percent of the time in 100 percent of the people? No. Some people are allergic to corn, some to wheat, to nuts, to strawberries, and other food substances. I have treated people brought to hospital emergency rooms after eating very innocent foods, such as nuts or corn: these people were suffering very severe allergic reactions. Does that mean we should ban strawberries, corn, wheat, nuts, and everything else someone is allergic to? Not at all. Among the millions of people in this country there is a certain measure of biochemical individuality to take into account.

### I've Heard That L-DOPA and L-Tyrosine Can Raise Your Blood Pressure. Will DLPA Raise Your Blood Pressure, Too?

Let me begin by saying that in published studies of DL- and D-phenylalanine use in human patients, blood pressure did not rise (when monitored). As for L-DOPA and L-tyrosine; both of these substances are converted into neurotransmitters in the brain and in peripheral nerves. Two of these neurotransmitters, norepinephrine (NE) and epinephrine (E), are found in nerve cells which regulate blood pressure. But there does not seem to be a simple relationship between amino acid intake and blood pressure. For example, several studies in experimental animals have shown that very large amounts of L-tyrosine can *either raise or lower* blood pressure, depending on the starting conditions.[1] In one study, large amounts of L-tyrosine (100 mg/kg/day, or about 7 grams per day for an average person) were given to patients. The point was to see if these large amounts of L-tyrosine would effect neurotransmitter levels. Even at this high dosage level, there was no disturbance in neurotransmitter activity.

I've been asked by several doctors if DLPA could raise blood pressure. I point out that orally administered L-DOPA (a product of LPA metabolism) commonly causes a slight, temporary *reduction* of blood pressure. To those who wonder if L-phenylalanine will raise blood pressure, I reply this has not happened in DLPA studies, and that the amount of LPA consumed daily on the DLPA Program is small compared to the amounts of L-tyrosine used in the above-mentioned reports. And it is important to note that any *potential* selective effects of an individual amino acid on NE or E activity will be greatly reduced when it is taken *with* proteins (meals).

In summary, the evidence, and my clinical experience indicate there is no reason to fear that DLPA, when taken as a part of the DLPA Program, will cause elevated blood pressure. If, however, you have any reason to be concerned with your blood pressure, I recommend you have it checked frequently by your physician. Regular blood pressure checks are a good idea for everyone.

### Is DLPA Really Legal?

Yes. DLPA is 100 percent legal, and is sold in vitamin and health food stores across the country. DLPA is classified by the federal government as a "Nutrient/Dietary Supplement." If you are still in doubt, look at Title 21 of the 1983 edition of the *U.S. Code of Federal Regulations*. There, under Section 582.5590, you will see that DL-phenylalanine is on the federal government's GRAS (Generally Recognized As Safe) list.

# 14

# REFLECTIONS ON THE MIND, ENDORPHINS, AND THOUGHTS

Some time in the future, a healthy volunteer allows a blood sample to be drawn and checked for endorphin activity. Stepping into a quiet room, he spends an hour in silent thought. The hour completed, he once again has his blood drawn and measured. Endorphin activity has increased by 50 percent.

A medical fantasy? I don't think so. I believe we can increase our endorphin levels without DL-phenylalanine (DLPA). Instead, we can use the power of our mind.

The power of our mind? Increase endorphins in our nervous system just by thinking about it? Is it really possible? Yes!

In one of the first studies of its kind, Dr. John Lipman[1] and his collaborators in the Department of Anesthesiology and Biochemistry at the University of Tennessee Center For Health Sciences measured endorphin levels in the spinal fluid of 32 chronic pain patients. Then the patients were given a placebo. Fourteen of the patients reported pain relief, which is to be expected. As you remember, the placebo effect works 30 to 40 percent of the time because people *think* they are supposed to get better. But this is the amazing part:

Endorphin levels went up in these 14 people. The placebo did not raise their endorphins—their thoughts did. The placebo was a worthless sugar pill, but their thoughts were pure gold.

## MIRACLES?

As a medical doctor, I usually see the other side of the coin, the many people who "think" themselves sick, not well. I have treated many people who got sick because they filled their minds with negative thoughts, setting up the mental conditions favoring disease. I am not saying that everyone who is sick "thought" themselves sick—but many of the patients I have seen had poor Mental Blueprints to thank for their illness. Centuries ago it was written:

"The thing which I greatly feared has come unto me, and that which I was afraid of is come unto me."

—Job 3:25

This Biblical passage describes what I see in the hospitals and in my office; disease caused by fear, anxiety, anger, and all the other negative feelings.

"The thing which I greatly feared." What does that mean? For modern people, the thing which we greatly fear is failure, rejection, loss of finanical security, and loss of personal security. And as I pointed out in chapter 3, filing our heads with these negative thoughts undermines our physical health. With poor Mental Blueprints and poor health, that which you greatly fear is very likely to happen.

Working in the "front lines" of medicine, I saw a great deal of pain and death in the hospital wards, emergency rooms, intensive care units, and coronary care units. I saw many patients, who, when told they had only a short time to live, would just lie down and die. The doctor gave them the bad news, and they meekly put this bad news into their mind and died.

But I also saw many patients who refused to give up. Despite the so-called "realistic judgment" of squadrons of specialists, these seriously ill patients refused to roll over and die. They shut the negative, "realistic" news out of their minds and kept their Mental Blueprints pure: And they recovered!

As a young doctor I was very "scientific" and "realistic." I went by the book. If someone had a particular disease, he or she had so much time to live and that was that. But through the years

I learned something about, well, I guess you'd call it faith. I saw patients with faith in themselves, with faith in their ability to recover, and most important, *with a burning desire to live*. And you know what? These are the ones who were more likely to live.

Miracles? If by miracles you mean an unexpected, unexplained happening contrary to the laws of nature, contrary to our "realism"—then yes, they were miracles.

I could not explain them, but I was convinced these miracles were a psychological phenomenon: The mind was telling the body what to do. As I began to study the effects of stress on people, I saw that there was indeed a very strong biochemical link between the mind and the rest of the body. The mind is literally able to make the rest of the body sick—or very healthy.

## FROM THOUGHTS TO BIOCHEMISTRY

Back in the early part of this century, Walter Cannon, M.D., a great physiologist at Harvard, described how threats to our well-being, real or imagined, trigger the "fight or flight" response. This well-accepted phenomenon describes how a threat to a person's body, ego, well-being, or security is automatically transformed into a hurly-burly of biochemical activity preparing the person to either fight, or run, for his or her life.

The "fight or flight" response is a good way to deal with sudden danger. But we turn the response on too often for no good reason at all. How do we turn it on? All it takes is negative thoughts. All you have to do is get angry at someone. All you have to do is put yourself, or someone else down. All it takes is a few negative thoughts to set "negative" chemicals to work on your body.

What happens when negative thoughts cover your Mental Blueprints and trigger the "fight or flight" response over and over again, for no reason? Tidal waves of chemicals speed through the body, stressing one body system after another, literally killing them with stress and overwork.

In times of danger these chemicals may be necessary to save your life. At other times the chemicals can kill you. A small amount of these chemicals energize you, give you enthusiasm and drive. Too many of these chemicals set you up for disease and death.

What about depression? Is there a biochemical description of depression as well? Your "feeling brain," the limbic system, responds to threats to your security by instructing the hypothalamus, pituitary gland, and adrenal glands to withdraw, to slow down and conserve by withholding stimulating hormones. You lose energy, your sexual and maternal drives diminish, your appetite suffers, you feel subordinate, have less desire to extend yourself, and so on. This can kick off a downward spiral of threats to your security, feelings of helplessness, depression, loss of control, more depression, and on and on.

## BETTER LIVING THROUGH YOUR BRAIN

Through your brain and body chemistry you can have better, or worse living. The choice is yours. If the patients in the placebo study could use the power of their minds to raise their endorphin levels, so can you.

Let's see what some of our teachers and philosophers have said about the power of the mind:

> "If your eye is pure, there will be sunshine in your soul. But if your eye is clouded with evil thoughts and desires, you are in deep spiritual darkness. And oh, how deep that darkness can be."

> —Matthew, 6:22, 23—*The Living Bible*

What Matthew means is that if you develop the habit of looking for the best in yourself and in others, if you seek out happiness, your brain will make the "right" kinds and proportions of "happy chemicals," and you will be happy. But if you write "anger" and "unhappiness" all over your Mental Blueprint, what begins as a "spiritual darkness" will soon become physical illness.

Ralph Waldo Emerson told us that a person's life is what he thinks all day long. Positive, happy thinking equals a positive, happy life. Marcus Aurelius, a Roman emperor, said the same thing many centuries earlier: "A man's life is what his thoughts make of it." In a more poetic vein, the emperor also said: "The soul is dyed the color of your thoughts."

## RENEWAL

"Be you transformed by the renewing of your mind."

—Romans, 12:2

The people in the placebo study were transformed by the power of their minds. Their positive thoughts, "I am going to get better!" were reflected in increased endorphin activity in their central nervous system. The endorphins blocked their pain and lifted their spirits. They were transformed by the renewing of their minds, transformed by their endorphins.

I am not saying that if you tell yourself "everything is wonderful" you will suddenly make a million dollars, marry the man or woman of your dreams, and invent a better mousetrap. What I am saying is this:

Your mind has a profound influence over the rest of your body. Your mind can make or break you. The constant stream of thoughts and ideas lodged in your brain—good and bad—are not simply floating aimlessly around. Their very presence is affecting your biochemistry, determining the composition and ratios of your body chemistry.

You can be—you are!—your best doctor. You do not need a medical degree or a stethoscope. All you have to do is take up your "mental pen" and fill your Mental Blueprints with strong, positive thoughts. Your body will do the rest.

Begin by forgiving and forgetting. Get rid of all the little gripes and grudges and grievances. Forget about what this one or that one did to you six years ago, forget about past failures. Wipe your Mental Blueprint clean and start again.

"This one thing I do, forgetting those things which are behind and reaching forth unto those things which are before me, I press toward the mark . . ."

—Philippians, 3:13,14

Too many people can't sleep at night because they remember all the little hurts and wrongs done to them by others; or worse, done to them by themselves. Constantly dredging up these unhappy thoughts causes high voltage chemicals to be "dumped" inappropriately into your body. When you find yourself dwelling on the unhappy thoughts of past deeds and what could have been, remember that you are upsetting the biochemistry of your brain and body.

Make the biochemistry of your brain a happy biochemistry: Forgive and Forget. Tell yourself: Right now I forgive myself for any failure or mistep I might have taken. I forgive myself freely and altogether. In forgiving myself I forgive everyone else in my life who I believed might have wronged me. *Now I am free* to go forward and have what I want in life: Health, Happiness, Love, Success, and Prosperity.

## BIOCHEMICAL RENEWAL

Wiping the negative thoughts from your mind will clean up the worst biochemical sewer. Having done that, replenish your biochemical storehouses with endorphins, the "happy chemicals." You know how to do it—the same way the placebo patients did. Just believe. Believe in yourself, believe in the power of your mind, and believe in your ability to succeed.

We read in the Scriptures that Moses told the Children of Israel:

> "Behold I set before you life and death, blessing and curse. Therefore, choose life."
>
> —Deuteronomy, 30:19

Choose Life, Health, and Love.

# APPENDIX I

# DLPA Safety Studies

I cannot emphasize enough that DLPA is a very safe, nutritional substance your body is well equipped to metabolize. Study after study has shown that, aside from a feeling of "excitement" in a very few people, DLPA has no adverse side effects.

Both the D- and DL-forms of phenylalanine have been administered in large single doses to human subjects in several reported studies, without apparent toxic effects. For example, Jervis[1] administered fairly large doses (5 gm) of the L-, D-, and DL-forms of phenylalanine to a male subject. While no toxic effects were observed, the administration of D-phenylalanine resulted in the excretion of larger amounts of phenylpyruvic acid than either the DL- or L-forms (which yielded equal amounts of phenylpyruvic acid). Wang and Waisman[2] conducted phenylalanine tolerance tests (using DLPA) in sixteen normal subjects. The dosage level was 0.2 gm per kilogram body weight. (Such a dosage level would result in 10.0-14.0 gm dosages in 50-70 kg subjects, respectively.) No toxic effects were observed. Levine et al[3] studies phenylalanine metabolism in eight premature infants. Dosages ranging from .50 to 9.0 gm per day of DL-phenylalanine were administered orally as part of an experiment designed to study tyrosine formation from dietary phenylalanine. It was found that L-tyrosine was not capable of replacing DLPA in the diet. No toxic effects of DL-phenylalanine were noted, although the high doses resulted in the formation of excessive amounts of L-tyrosine, which were excreted in the urine (this is the primary metabolic product of L-phenylalanine in all mammalian species).

In a study of human dietary needs for essential amino acids, Bassett et al[4] supplied essential amino acids parenterally to a patient recovering from abdominal surgery. Included in the study were three different amino acid formulas which contained either five, ten, or 11.1 gm of DLPA (six of the ten amino acids studied were supplied in the DL-form).

These dietary solutions were administered in either two or three equally divided injections during the day. It was noted that:

> Tolerance for the amino acid solutions was high. Its limits were not reached during this experiment, although the rates of injections used were more rapid than any recorded for protein-digest solutions with freedom from clinical disturbance. No rise in body temperature as a result of the injection was observed.

Numerous physiologic variables were monitored, including plasma chlorides, carbon dioxide "combining power" of the blood, nitrogen balance and body weight. No abnormal or toxic effects were noted. It was concluded that essential amino acids could be provided in their purified (and in some cases racemic) form "without any clinical disturbance, and with satisfaction of the requirements of nitrogen equilibrium and formation of body protein."

Madden and Whipple[5] administered amino acid solutions containing 6.9 to 11.1 gm per day of DLPA (and five other racemic amino acids) to three patients over long periods of time (from thirty to seventy-five days). Routes of administration included oral, subcutaneous and intravenous. The results showed that nitrogen balance could be suitably maintained in all cases. Furthermore, the authors stated that "no evidence of serious or persistent injury has ever been noted after any of hundreds of injections into animals and man using the materials (which included relatively large amounts of DL-phenylalanine) here studied." They further commented that the data gives "no evidence that the unnatural (D-) isomers of the amino acids are toxic and some are probably used in the body". Madden *et al*[6] confirmed these results in two additional patients during preoperative and postoperative periods. (The patients exhibited normal healing following surgery.) Using the same amino acid solutions as in their previous study (see footnote five), the authors reported "no toxicity to the unnatural isomers of seven essential amino acids was demonstrated," and, in fact, normal healing processes were observed during the weeks when the solutions were administered.

The table below summarizes the results of studies in human subjects:

## LACK OF TOXICITY OF PHENYLALANINE ISOMERS IN HUMANS

| Dosage (grams) | Isomeric Form | Conditions | Single(S) or Divided (D) Dose | Unusual Physiologic Reactions? | Toxic Effect? | See Footnote Number |
|---|---|---|---|---|---|---|
| 5.0 | D- | Metabolic Study | S | No | No | 1 |
| 10–14* | DL- | Phenylalanine Tolerance Test | S | No | No | 2 |
| .50–9.0 | DL- | Metabolism In Infants | D | No | No | 3 |
| 5–11.1 | DL- | Parenteral** Nutrition (post-operative) | D | No | No | 4 |
| 6.9–11.5 | DL- | Parenteral Nutrition | D | No | No | 5 |
| 1.1–2.4 | DL- | Dietary Requirement | D | No | No | 7 |
| 5.4 | DL- | Nutritional Research | D | No | No | 8 |
| 4.58 | DL- | Nutritional Research | D | No | No | 9 |
| 4.0 | D- | Acupuncture Enhancement | S | No | No | 10 |

\* Estimate based on .20 gm/kg dosage level in subject weighing approximately 50–70 kg.
\*\* Intravenous

195

# APPENDIX II

# Treatment of Depression With DLPA and DPA

Both D- and DL-phenylalanine have been used in the treatment of depression since 1974 when Yaryura-Tobias et al[1] administered 100 mg of DL- or D-phenylalanine per day to patients exhibiting symptoms of endogenous depression. Ten of the 15 patients showed a substantial improvement within two weeks after treatment began. The authors observed "no toxic effects" and found that in the patients who responded favorably to treatment, "no further medication" was necessary. And, in patients requiring further treatment, DPA and DLPA "enhanced the action of tricyclic antidepressants."

This study was motivated by a growing body of literature indicating that beta-phenylethylamine (PEA) was involved in a multitude of central nervous system processes generally believed to mediate states of arousal and activation. PEA is structurally very similar to amphetamine, and evokes similar behavior patterns (such as increased arousal). Fischer et al[2] were among the first to propose a link between PEA and depression in 1968 when they reported decreased urinary levels of PEA in depressed patients. While normal subjects eliminated a mean of 35.5 ug/1, depressed patients had immeasurably low levels. Using more sophisticated assay methods in a later study, Fischer et al[3] collected 24-hour urine samples (pooled) from normal and depressed patients. They found the endogenous depression patients had significantly decreased basal levels of PEA (mean urinary elimination of 114 ug%) compared to normals (mean of 336%). Patients with secondary and atypical depressions did not show decreased levels. Treatment of endogenously depressed patients with either chlorimipramine or desimipramine (75 mg daily) led to increased urinary PEA and reductions in depressive symptomologies. Concomitant with this clinical work were reports that both L- and D-phenylalanine induced increases in brain levels of PEA.[4] Unfortunately, PEA assays were not performed on the patients in the Yaryura-Tobias *et al* study, so we cannot say that increased PEA synthesis or availability was responsible for the apparent beneficial effects of D- and DL-phenylalanine in this study. Still, this study suggested a therapeutic role for phenylalanine in depression.

In the year following the Yaryura-Tobias report, Fisher *et al*[5] reported on treating 23 patients presenting typical symptoms of endogenous depression with either D- or DL-phenylalanine. Doses varied from 50-200 mg daily. Although these patients had not previously responded to antidepressant drugs, a "complete euthymia" was noted in 17 of the 23 within 13 days. While "no important adverse reaction was observed" in the participants, there were some episodes of transient headaches and vertigo. It is not known whether these problems were related to the phenylalanine or not.

Spatz *et al*[6] assessed the effects of DPA on 11 patients' "clinical state" (a behavioral rating scale) and urinary PEA levels (pooled 24 hour samples). Seven of the patients were classified as endogenous depressives, 4 as atypical. All patients received a twice-daily dose which increased from 50 mg/dose to 100 mg/dose over a 15 day period. PEA levels rose dramatically in 10 of the 11 patients, and tended to drop when treatment was stopped. A marked improvement was noted in most patients. It's interesting to note that the patient enjoying the least improvement ("slight improvement") was the one whose PEA levels did not climb dramatically. The authors suggested that decreased PEA availability in the CNS may play a causative role in mental depression, and that the antidepressant effects of DPA are due to its preferential decarboxylation to PEA. This study linked oral DPA administration in humans to increased PEA excretion and an apparently related improvement in behavioral state.

Beckman *et al*[7] used more rigorous, standardized procedures to assess the behavioral state of 20 depressed patients as they studied the antidepressant properties of DLPA. The International Classification of Diseases scoring system was used to classify 10 of the 20 as monopolar endogenous depressives, and 6 as involutional endogenous depressives. 25 mg DLPA tablets were give to the patients three times a day. Patients received no other antidepressant medication during the treatment period. Neurologic, psychopathological, and somatic changes were assessed using the AMP system, the Hamilton Depression Scale, a self-rating scale, and a global clinical impression. These tests were administered to each patient by at least two psychiatrists several times during the course of the study. Within 20 days 8 patients enjoyed complete euthymia, 4 showed a marked improvement, 4 demonstrated a moderate improvement, and 4 were nonresponsive. DLPA was most effective against endogenous depression (monopolar and involutional); 80 percent of these patients responded favorably. EEG, EKG, blood pressure and body temperature were monitored daily through the study, but no abnormal activity associated with the DLPA were noted. (One patient experienced polytopic extrasystoles on one day and several patients experienced transient headaches. The conditions abated spontaneously without discontinuing treatment.) In their comments, the authors referred to Fisher *et al*[8] and others who reported that only a certain percent of depressed patients excrete decreased levels of PEA, implying that only this portion of the patient population would respond to phenylalanine.

Beckman *et al*[9] replicated these findings in a double-blind controlled study in 1979. Following a 2-to-3-day placebo washout period, patients were given either 150-200 mg/day DLPA or the same range of imipramine (a tricyclic antidepressant). Analysis of patient scores on the Hamilton Depression Scale and the AMP classification system over the course of the study indicated that both compounds exerted significant antidepressant effects, and that the antidepressant effects of the two treatments were indistinguishable. Adverse effects were minimal in both groups, but the DLPA group experienced fewer autonomic disturbances (dryness of the mouth, constipation, micturation problems, etc.). Heller[10] conducted a large scale DPA/depression study using several groups of patients with varying diagnoses. Following a 7 day washout period, an open design was used in administering 100-400 mg/day for periods ranging from 2 to 6 months. Hamilton's, Zung's, and Beck's rating scales for depressive symptomologies were used to determine the patients' clinical states. Within 60 days of beginning treatment, approximately 95 percent of the 370 endogenous depression patients were felt to have achieved a normal affective state, or to have shown improvement. Eighty-five percent of the 47 neurotically depressed patients also achieved a normal affective state or enjoyed improvement. (This is according to the author's own rating scale. The results of the other behavioral rating scales was not reported.) Heller also conducted a double-blind, controlled study comparing the efficacy of DPA to that of imipramine. Sixty patients were divided into two groups and given 100 mg/day (50 mg twice a day) of either the amino acid or the tricyclic. These endogenous depression patients were given DPA or imipramine for 15 days, placebo for 5 days, and their original medication through day 30. Within 15 days, 60 percent of the D-phenylalanine group, and 30 percent of the imipramine group were considered to have reached a normal affective state. By the fifth day of placebo administration, these figures had dropped to 6 percent and 3 percent, respectively.

Treatment was resumed, and by day 30, 66 percent of the D-phenylalanine group and 43 percent of the imipramine group were again classified as having a normal affective state. Statistical comparisons were not performed on the data, but the DPA group appears to have enjoyed substantially greater improvement than the imipramine group did. The urinary PEA levels of 7 patients in each of the two groups were monitored as part of the study. D-phenylalanine led to a mean increase of 1300 percent in urinary PEA levels, compared to about a 750 percent increase with imipramine. Urinary PEA levels returned almost all the way back to normal during the placebo period. The data suggests a relationship between DPA, PEA levels, and patient status, providing strong support for the involvement of PEA in the antidepressant actions of DPA (and imipramine, for that matter). As did the other investigators, Heller reported that "no side effects or toxic reactions were observed with treatment with D-phenylalanine."

The studies I've reviewed here indicate that both D- and DL-phenylalanine have substantial antidepressant actions, especially in patients with endogenous depression. The mechanisms by which this is accomplished are not certain, but several studies apparently show a significant relationship between clinical assessment and urinary PEA levels.

In spite of the fact that L-phenylalanine is the principal precursor for PEA synthesis, it has been proposed that the D-isomer is responsible for phenylalanine's antidepressant actions. Data collected by Spatz and Spatz[11] suggests a possible basis for the differing antidepressant effects of the two isomers. Spatz and Spatz studied the production of PEA in rat brain during a 48 hour period following the intraperitoneal injection of D- or L-phenylalanine. They found that at dosages of 5 mg/kg and 100 mg/kg, DPA induced a greater mean increase of PEA (except at one point). The difference may be due to the fact that LPA is utilized by peripheral tissue in biosynthetic processes (such as protein synthesis), while more of the D-isomer is allowed to reach the brain. The authors concluded that such an effect may form the basis for the greater antidepressant effectiveness of DPA compared to LPA. And in the report of his studies, Heller[12] noted that "When low doses of D- and L-phenylalanine are injected into rats, both raise the brain PEA content but the effects of D-phenylalanine are significantly more effective than those of L-phenylalanine."

A possible explanation for Spatz and Spatz's data is offered by the work of Borison et al.[13] Their experiments suggest that DPA is directly decarboxylated to PEA. Because of the presence of the D-isomer, DLPA would be expected to exert its actions via the same mechanisms. This, in conjunction with the apparently significant relationship of PEA levels and depressive symptomology, offers support for a significant role for PEA in DLPA and DPA's antidepressant actions.

Leaving PEA aside for the moment, let's look at the possible role endorphins play in the antidepressant effects of DPA and DLPA. We know that both these phenylalanine forms inhibit enzymes which degrade endogenous opioids, and that exogenous opioids (narcotics) have considerable euphorogenic properties. Thus, it's not unreasonable to propose a role for the endorphins. Numerous published reports support this suggestion. Angst et al[14] gave synthetic human beta-endorphin to two unipolar and four bipolar depressed patients. Four of the six experienced a pronounced antidepressant effect which lasted several hours. Kline et al[15] reported antidepressant effects in 2 of 3 unipolar depressives given synthetic human beta-endorphin intravenously in a single-blind study. Krebs and Roubicek[16] observed dramatic antidepressant effects in 3 of 4 depressed patients who received the peptidase-resistant analogue of methionine-enkephalin, FK 33-824. And, in a controlled study, Gerner et al[17] administered either beta-endorphin or saline (i.v.) to 10 depressed patients. The researchers found a significant positive change in overall patient rating among those given the endorphin, compared to placebo.

The studies reviewed in this appendix suggest that DPA and DLPA may exert their antidepressant effects both through PEA and through protection of endorphins.

# APPENDIX III

# Treatment Of Arthritis With DLPA and DPA

The publication of Dr. Seymour Ehrenpreis' 1978 study[1] on DPA and pain suggested that D-phenylalanine might be an effective treatment for arthritis. One participant in this study had osteoarthritis in the fingers and thumbs of both hands which had lasted 5 years. The patient experienced "excellent relief" of pain and a reduction of joint stiffness. A second patient with rheumatoid arthritis of the left knee and osteoarthritis of the hands (of several years duration) enjoyed "considerable relief." Subsequent clinical investigations have shown that D-phenylalanine and DL-phenylalanine exert powerful antiinflammatory actions which often produce dramatic increases in joint flexibility. In a 1982 review, Ehrenpreis[2] noted "that of the chronic pain patients treated with D-phenylalanine, those who responded best were experiencing some kind of inflammation."

The precise manner in which DPA and DLPA reduce inflammation is uncertain. In an earlier investigation[3] it was found that enkephalins and prostaglandins are mutually antagonistic modulators of pain perception. As phenylalanine "protects" endorphins, it may retard the inflammatory actions of prostaglandins by making more enkephalin available. Ferreira and Nakamura[4] have studied the effects of enkephalin on inflammation-induced hyperalgesia produced by prostaglandin $E_2$ ($PGE_2$) and carageenin. They found that methionine-enkephalin and morphine "produced similar analgesic effects" when injected into animal paws inflamed by carageenin. The researchers stated that methionine-enkephalin was "approximately 100 times more potent" than lidocaine. The methods used in this study suggest a peripheral (as opposed to central) mode of action for methionine-enkephalin. This supports the argument that enkephalins of adrenal origin play a role in analgesic processes. The authors speculated that the peripheral analgesic effects of methionine-enkephalin may occur directly at the nociceptors themselves. (The peptidase-resistant enkephalin analogue "BW 180d" also greatly reduced hyperalgesic inflammatory responses induced by $PGE_2$ or carageenin.) It may be that the secretion of pituitary beta-endorphin and adrenal enkephalins are an essential component of the body's primary antiinflammatory response. Guillemin et al[5] have demonstrated the co-secretion of ACTH and beta-endorphin from the anterior pituitary, and it is generally accepted that the mobilization of endogenous opioids is an integral part of the response to stress.[6] But unlike the corticosteriods, endorphins retard inflammation and elicit analgesia. Pituitary beta-endorphin, like ACTH, may also stimulate synthesis of corticosteriods in the adrenal gland.[7]

The work of Oliveras et al[8] suggests that an endorphin deficiency may be responsible for the hyperalgesic state found in arthritis. These researchers demonstrated that naloxone (the endorphin antagonist) produces a significantly greater hyperalgesic response in rats suffering from chronic arthritis than it does in controls. Preliminary research (see reference 2) indicates that arthritis patients might have abnormally low levels of endorphins in their synovial fluid. Dr. Charles Denko[9] has found low levels of endorphins in the blood of patients with several types of arthritis.

The various studies suggest the endorphins are involved in the symptomology, and possibly the etiology, of arthritic syndromes. It may be that such states are due to an endorphin deficiency caused by:

1. impaired secretion of beta-endorphin from the pituitary and/or reduced secretion of enkephalin from the adrenal gland;
2. reduced biosynthesis of endorphin/enkephalin precursors in the pituitary and/or adrenal gland;
3. overactivity of endorphin-degrading enzymes in the synovial fluid or adrenal gland.

If this is the case, the use of D- or DL-phenylalanine in arthritis would counteract the problem more effectively than any currently available therapy.

# FOOTNOTES

## CHAPTER 1
1. Pert, C.R., and S.H. Snyder, 1973. Opiate receptor: Demonstration in nervous tissue. *Science* 179: 1011–14.

## CHAPTER 2
1. "Unlocking Pain's Secrets." June 11, 1984. *Time* magazine, p.59.

## CHAPTER 3
1. Fox, A. 1983. Aloe Vera's $B_{12}$—A new discovery. *Total Health* 5(4), pp.48–51.

## CHAPTER 4
1. Baldessarini, R.J. 1975. Biogenic amine hypothesis in affective disorders. In *The nature and treatment of depression,* eds. F.F. Flack and S.C. Draghi, New York: Wiley, pp. 347–85.

2. Yaryura-Tobias, J.A., B. Heller, H. Spatz, and E. Fischer. 1974. Phenylalanine for endogenous depression. *Journal of Orthomolecular Psychiatry* 3(2), pp. 80–81.

3. Fisher, E., B. Heller, M. Nachon, and N. Spatz. 1975. Therapy of depression by phenylalanine. *Arzneim Forsch.* 251: 132.

4. Beckmann, H., M.A. Strauss,, and E. Ludolph. 1977. DL-phenylalanine in depressed patients: An open study. *J. Neural Trans.* 41: 123–24.

5. Heller, B. 1978. Pharmacological and clinical effects of DL-phenylalanine in depression and Parkinson's disease. In *Modern pharmacology-toxicology, noncatecholic phenylethylamines,* Part 1, eds. A.D. Mosnaim and M.E. Wolfe, New York: Marcel Dekker, pp. 397–417.

6. Ibid.

7. Beckmann, H., D. Athen, M. Oheanu, and R. Zimmer. 1979. DL-phenylalanine versus imipramine: a double-blind controlled study. *Arch. Psychiat. Nervenkr.* 227: 49–58.

8. Gerner, R.H., D.A. Gorelick, D.H. Catlin, and C.H. Li. 1982. Behavioral effects of beta-endorphin in depression and schizophrenia. In

*Endorphins and opiate antagonists in psychiatric research, clinical implications,* New York: Plenum, pp. 257–70.

9. Kline, N.S., C.H. Li, H.E. Lehmann, A. Lajtha, E. Laske, and T. Cooper. 1977. Beta-endorphin induced changes in schizophrenic and depressed patients. *Arch. Gen. Psychiatry,* 34: 1111–13; Angst, J., V. Autenreith, F. Brem, M. Koukkou, H. Meyer, H.H. Stassen, and V. Storck. 1980. Preliminary results of treatment with beta-endorphin in depression. In *Endorphins in mental health research,* eds. E. Usdin, W.E. Bunney, and M.S. Kline. London: Macmillan, pp. 518–28; Gerner, R.H., D.H. Catlin, D.A. Gorelick, K.K. Hui, and C.H. Li. 1980. Beta-endorphin. Intravenous infusion causes behavioral change in psychiatric inpatients. *Arch. Gen. Psychiatry,* 37: 642–47; Ruther, E., G. Jungkunz, and N. Nedopil. 1981. Clinical effects of the synthetic analogue of methionine enkephalin, FK 33-824. *Third World Congress of Biological Psychiatry,* Stockholm (abstract).

10. Jakubovic, A. 1982. Psychoactive agents and enkephalin degradation. In *Endorphins and opiate antagonists in psychiatric research,* eds. N.S. Shah and A.G. Donald. New York: Plenum, pp. 89–97.

11. Sabelli, H., and A.D. Mosnaim. 1974. Phenylethylamine hypothesis of affective behavior. *Am. J. Psychiatry,* 131: 695–99.

12. Spatz, H., B. Heller, M. Nachon, and E. Fischer. 1975. Effects of D-phenylalanine on clinical picture and phenylethylaminuria in depression. *Biol. Psychiatry,* 10(2): 235–39; Heller, B. 1978. Pharmacological and clinical effects of D-phenylalanine in depression and Parkinson's disease, In *Modern pharmacology-toxicology, noncatecholic phenylethylamines,* Part 1, eds. A.D. Mosnaim and M.E. Wolf. New York: Marcel Dekker, pp. 397–417; Fisher, E., B. Heller, M. Nachon, and N. Spatz. 1975. Therapy of depression by phenylalanine. *Arzneim-Forsch.* 251: 132; Beckman, Strauss, and Ludolph. op. cit.; Yaryura-Tobias, J.A., B. Heller, H. Spatz, and E. Fisher. 1974. Phenylalanine for endogenous depression. *J. Ortho. Psychiat.* 3(2): 80–81.

13. Klein, D.F. and M. Leibowitz. December 1979. "Affective Disorders: Special Clinical Forms," Psychiatric Clinics of North America.

**CHAPTER 6**

1. Arthritis Foundation. 19. *Arthritis: Basic Facts.* Arthritis Foundation, Public Education Department, Atlanta, Georgia. Publication No. 4001/6–83.

2. Ehrenpreis, S., R.C. Balagot, S. Myles, C. Advocate, and J.E.

Comaty. 1978. Further studies on the analgesic activity of D-phenyla-lanine (DPA) in mice and humans. *Endogenous and exogenous opiate agonists and antagonists,* ed. by E. Leony Way, Elmsford, N.Y.: Pergammon, pp. 379–82.

3. Ehrenpreis, S., J. Greenberg, K. Kubota, and S. Myles. 1981. Analgesic properties of D-phenylalanine, bacitracin, and puromycin in mice: Relationship to inhibition of enkephalinase and beta-endorphi-nase. *Advances in endorphins and exogenous opioids: Proceedings of the international narcotic research conference,* eds. H. Takagi and E. J. Simon. Tokyo: Kodansha, pp. 279–81.

4. Balagot, R., S. Ehrenpreis, K. Kubota, and J. Greenberg. 1983. Analgesia in mice and humans by D-phenylalanine: Relation to inhibition of enkephalin degradation and enkephalin levels. *Advances in Pain Research and Therapy* 5: pp. 289–93. Eds. J. J. Bonica *et al*. Raven Press, N.Y.

5. Ferreira, S. and M. Nakamura. 1979. II-Prostaglandin hyperalge-sia: The peripheral analgesic activity of morphine, enkephalins and opioid antagonists. *Prostaglandins* 18: 191–200.

**CHAPTER 8**

1. Laversen, N.H., and E. Stukane. 1983. *Premenstrual syndrome and you*. New York: Simon and Schuster, p. 171.

2. Ibid.

3. Reid, R. H., and S.S.C. Yen. 1981. Premenstrual syndrome. *Am. J. obstetrics and gynecology* 139: 85–104.

4. Halbreich, U., and J. Endicott. 1981. Possible involvement of endorphin withdrawal or imbalance in specific premenstrual syndromes and postpartum depression. *Medical Hypothesis* 7: 1045–58.

5. Bruni, J.F., D. VanVugt, S. Marshall, and J. Meites. 1977. Effects of naloxone, morphine and methionine-enkephalin on serum prolactin, leutenizing hormone, follicle-stimulating hormone, thyroid-stimulating hormone and growth hormone. *Life Sci* 21: 461. Dupont, A. *et al*. 1982. Relationship of opiate peptides to neuroendocrine functions. In: *Endorphins and Opiate Antagonists in Psychiatric Research*. Edited by N.S. Shah and A.G. Donald. Plenum Medical, NY, pp. 99–126. Wehrenberg, W.B., S.L. Wardlaw, A.G. Frantz, and M. Ferin, 1982. Beta-endorphin in hypophyseal portal blood: Variations throughout the menstrual cycle. *Endocrinology* III: pp. 879–82.

6. Billig, Harvey E. Jr., and C. Arthur Spaulding, Jr. 1947. Hy-perinsulism of menses. *Industrial Medicine* (July) pp. 336–39.

## CHAPTER 10

1. Mayer, D.J., D.D. Price, A. Rafii. 1977. Antagonism of acupuncture analgesia in man by the narcotic antagonist naloxone. *Brain Research* 121: 368–72.

2. Clement-Jones, V., L. McLoughlin, S. Tomlin, G.M. Besser, L.H. Rees, and H.L. Wen. 1980. Increased beta-endorphin but not met-enkephalin levels in human cerebrospinal fluid after acupuncture or recurrent pain. *Lancet* 2: 946–49.

3. Nakano, S., and E. Ikezono. 1981. Effects of electroacupuncture on the levels of endorphins and substances P in human lumbar CSF. In *Advances in endogenous and exogenous opioids*, eds. J. Takagi and E.J. Simon. Tokyo: Kodansha-Elsevier, pp. 312–14.

4. Cheng, R.S.S., and B. Pomeranz. 1979. Correlation of genetic differences in endorphin systems with analgesic effects of D-amino acids in mice. *Brain Research* 177: 583–87. Cheng, R. S., and B. Pomeranz. 1980. A combined treatment with D-amino acids and electroacupuncture produces a greater analgesia than either treatment alone; naloxone reverses these effects. *Pain* 8: 231–36.

5. Hyodo, M., T. Kitade and E. Hosoka. 1983. Study on the enhanced analgesic effect induced by phenylalanine during acupuncture analgesia in humans. *Advances in Pain Research and Therapy* 5: 577–82.

## CHAPTER 11

1. Villet, B. 1978. Opiates of the mind. *The Atlantic* (June), 82–89.

2. Pert, C.R., and S.H. Snyder. 1973. Opiate receptor: Demonstration in nervous tissue. *Science 179:* 1011–14.

3. Kosterlitz, H.W., S.J. Paterson, and L.E. Robson. 1981. Opioid peptides and their receptors. In *Advances in Pharmacology and Therapeutics 2, Vol. 1: CNS Pharmacology Neuropeptides.* Edited by H. Yoshida, Y. Hagihara, and S. Ebashi. Pergamon, New York, pp. 3–13.

4. Hughes, J. 1975. Isolation of an endogenous compound from the brain with pharmacological properties similar to morphine. *Brain Res.* 88: 295–308. Hughes, J., H.W. Kosterlitz, and F.M. Leslie. 1974. Proceedings: Assessment of the agonist and antagonist activities of narcotic analgesic drugs by means of the mouse Vas deferens. *British Journal of Pharmacology* 51: 139–40. Hughes, J., T.W. Smith, H.W. Kosterlitz, L.A. Fothergill, B.A. Morgan, and H.R. Morris. 1975. Identification of two related pentapeptides from the brain with potent opiate agonist activity. *Nature* 258: 577–79.

5. Hambrook, J.M., F.A. Morgan, M.J. Rance, and C.F.C. Smith. 1976. Mode of deactivation of the enkephalins by rat and human plasma and rat brain homogenates. *Nature* 262: 282–85.

6. Dewey, W.L. 1982. Structure-activity relationships. In *Endorphins: Chemistry, physiology, pharmacology and clinical relevance.* Eds. J.B. Malick and R.M. Bell. New York: Marcel Dekker, pp. 23–56.

7. Li, C.H., D. Yamashiro, L.F. Tseng, and H.H. Loh. 1977. Synthesis and analgesic activity of human beta-endorphin. *J. Med. Chem.* 20: 325–28.

8. Ibid; Loh, H.H., L.F. Tseng, E. Wei, and C.H. Li. 1976. Beta-endorphin as a potent analgesic agent. *Proc. Natl. Acad. Sci.* 73: 2895–96.

9. Goldstein, A., S. Tachibana, L.I. Lowrey, M. Hunkapiller, and L. Hood. 1979. Dynorphin-(1-13), an extraordinarily potent opioid peptide. *Proceedings of the national academy of sciences,* Washington, D.C. 76: 6666.

10. Catlin, D.H., K.K. Hui, H.H. Loh, and C.H. Li. 1977. Pharmacologic activity of beta-endorphin in man. *Commun. Psychopharmacol.* 1: 493–500.

11. Hosobuchi, Y., and C.H. Li. 1978. The analgesic activity of human beta-endorphin in man. *Commun. Psychopharmacol.* 2: 33–37.

12. Oyama, T., T. Jin, R. Yamaya, A. Matsuki, N. Ling, and R. Guillemin. 1981. Intrathecal use of beta-endorphin as a powerful analgesic agent in man. In *Advances in pharmacology and therapeutics II: Vol. 1, CNS Pharmacology of neuropeptides,* eds. H. Yoshida, Y. Hagihara, and S. Ebashi. Elmsford, N.Y.: Pergamon, pp. 39–43.

13. Levine, J.D., N.C. Gordon, R.T. Jones, and H.L. Fields. 1978. The narcotic antagonist naloxone enchances clinical pain. *Nature* 272: 826–27.

14. Buchsbaum, M.S., G.C. Davis, and W.E. Bunney. 1977. Naloxone alters pain perception and somatosensory evoked potentials in normal subjects. *Nature* 270: 620–22.

15. Terenius, L. and A. Whalstrom. 1975. Morphine-like ligand for opiate receptors in human CSF. *Life Sci.* 16: 1759–64.

16. Von Knorring, L., F. Johansson, and B.G. Almay. 1982. The importance of the endorphin systems in chronic pain patients. In *Endorphins and opiate antagonists in psychiatric research: Clinical implications.* Eds. N.S. Shah and A.G. Donald. New York: Plenum, pp. 407–26.

17. Panerai, A.E., A. Martini, D. Abbate, R. Villani, and G.

DeBęnedittis. 1983. Beta-endorphin, met-enkephalin and beta-lipotropin in chronic pain and electroacupuncture. *Advances in Pain Research and Therapy* 5: 543–47. Eds. J. J. Bonica *et al.* Raven Press, N.Y.

18. Genazzani, A.R., G. Nappi, F. Fachinetti, G. Micieli, F. Petraglia, G. Bono, C. Monittola, and F. Savoldi. 1984. Progressive impairment of CSF beta-endorphin levels in migraine sufferers. *Pain*: 127–33.

19. Anselmi, B., E. Baldi, F. Cascecci, and S. Salmon. 1980. Endogenous opioids in cerebrospinal fluid and blood in idiopathic headache sufferers. *Headache* 21: 294–99. Baldi, E., S. Salmon, B. Anselmi, A. Capellini, G. Capelli, A. Brocchi, and F. Sicuteri. 1982. Intermittent hypoendorphinemia in migraine attack. *Cephalagia* 2: 77–81.

20. Denko, C.W., J. Aponte, P. Gabriel, and M. Petricevic. 1982. Serum beta-endorphin in rheumatoid disorders. *Journal of Rheumatology* 9: 827–33.

## CHAPTER 12

1. Ehrenpreis, S., R.C.Balagot, J.E. Comaty, and S.B. Myles, 1978. Naloxone-reversible analgesia in mice produced by D-phenylalaline and hydro-cinnamic acid, inhibitors of carboxypeptidase A. *Advances in Pain Research and Therapy,* Vol 3, edited by J. J. Bonica *et al.* pp. 479–88. Raven Press, NY.

2. Ehrenpreis, S., R.C. Balagot, S. Myles, C. Advocate, and J.E. Comaty. 1978. Further studies on the analgesic activity of D-phenylalanine (DPA) in mice and humans. In: *Endogenous and exogenous opiate agonists and antagonists,* edited by E. Way, pp. 379–82, Pergamon Press, Elmsford, NY.

3. Donzelle, G., L. Bernard, R. Deumier, M. Lacome, M. Barre, M. Lanier, and M.B. Mourtade. 1981. Curing trial of complicated oncologic pain by D-phenylalanine. *Anesth. Analg.* (Paris) 38: 655–58.

4. Balagot, R., S. Ehrenpreis, K. Kubota, and J. Greenberg. 1983. Analgesia in mice and humans by D-phenylalanine: Relation to inhibition of enkephalin degradation and enkephalin levels. *Advances in Pain Research and Therapy* Vol 5, edited by J.J. Bonica et al. Raven Press, NY, pp. 289–93.

5. Ehrenpreis, S., J. Greenberg, K. Kubota, and S. Myles. 1981. Analgesic properties of D-phenylalanine, bacitracin and puromycin in mice: Relationship to inhibition of enkephalinase and beta-endorphinase. In *Advances in endogenous and exogenous opioids: Proceedings of the international narcotic research conference.* Eds. H. Takagi and E.J. Simon, Tokyo: Kodansha-Elsevier, pp. 279–81.

6. Balagot, R., *et al op. cit.*

7. Budd, K. 1983. Use of D-phenylalanine, and enkephalinase inhibitor, in the treatment of intractable pain. *Advances in Pain Research and Therapy* 5: 305–08. J. J. Bonica *et al*. Raven Press, N.Y.

8. Lehman, W. D., N. Theobald, R. Fisher, and H. C. Heinrich. 1983. Stereospecificity of phenylalanine plasma kinetics and hydroxylation in man following oral application. *Clinica Chimica Acta* 128: 181–98.

Tokuhisa, S., K. Saisu, K. Naruse, H. Yoshikawa, and S. Baba. 1981. Studies on phenylalanine metabolism by tracer technique. IV. Biotransformation of D-L-phenylalanine in man. *Chem Pharm Bull* 29: 514–18.

9. Rose, W.C. 1976. Amino acid requirements of man. *Nutrition Reviews* 34(10): 307–08.

Rose, W.C., D.T. Warner, and W.J. Haines. 1951. The amino acid requirements of man. The role of leucine and phenylalanine. *J. Biol Chem*. 193: 613–20.

Rose, W.C., B.E. Leach, M.J. Coon, and G.F. Lambert. 1955. The amino acid requirements of man. The phenylalanine requirement. *J. Biol Chem*. 213: 913–22.

10. Jacquet, Y.F., W.A. Klee, and D.G. Smyth.1978. Beta-endorphin: Modulation of acute tolerance and antagonism by endogenous brain systems. *Brain Research* 156: 396–401.

## CHAPTER 13

1. Sved, A.F., J.D. Fernstrom, and R.J. Wurtman. 1979. Tyrosine administration reduces blood pressure and enhances brain norepinephrine release in spontaneously hyperactive rats. *Proceedings of the National Academy of Sciences (Washington, D.C.)* 76(7): 3511-14.

Conlay, L.A., T.J. Maher, and R.J. Wurtman. 1981. Tyrosine increases blood pressure in hypotensive rats. *Science* 212: 559–60.

## CHAPTER 14

1. Lipman, J. J., B. E. Miller, K. S. Mays, W. C. North, S. Karkera, and W. L. Bryne. 1981. CSF endorphin levels in chronic pain patients before and after placebo pain relief. *Advances in endogenous and exogenous opioids: Proceedings of the international narcotic research conference,* eds. H. Takagi and E. J. Simon. Tokyo: Kodansha, pp. 315–17.

APPENDIX I

1. Jervis, G. A. 1938. Metabolic investigations of phenylpyruvic oligophernia. *J. Biol. Chem.* 126: 305–13.

2. Wang, H. L., and H. A. Waisman. 1967. Phenylalanine tolerance tests in patients with leukemia. *J. Lab. Clin. Med.* 57: 73–77.

3. Levine, S. Z., M. Dann, and E. Marples. 1943. A defect in the metabolism of tyrosine and phenylalanine in premature infants. III. Demonstration of the irreversible conversion of phenylalanine to tyrosine in the human organism. *J. Clin. Invest.* 22: 551–60.

4. Bassett, S. H., R. R. Woods, F. W. Shull, and S. C. Madden. 1944. Parenterally administered amino acids as a source of protein in man. *N. Eng. J. Med.* 230(4): 106–08.

5. Madden, S. C., and G. H. Whipple. 1946. Amino acids in the production of plasma protein and nitrogen balance. *Am. J. Med. Sci.* 211: 149–56.

6. Madden, S. C., S. H. Basset, J. H. Remington, F. J. C. Martin, R. R. Woods and F. W. Shull. 1946. Amino acids in therapy of disease. Parenteral and oral administrations compared. *Surg. Gynecol. and Ob.* 82: 131–43.

7. Rose, W. C., B. E. Leach, M. J. Coon, and G. F. Lambert. 1955. The amino acid requirements of man. The phenylalanine requirement. *J. Biol. Chem.* 213: 913–22.

8. Rose, W. C., M. C. Coon and F. Lambert. 1954. The amino acid requirements of man. VI. The role of caloric intake. *J. Biol. Chem.* 210: 331–42.

9. Ibid.

10. Hyodo, M., T. Kitade, and E. Hosoka. 1983. Study on the enhanced analgesic effect induced by phenylalanine during acupuncture analgesia in humans. *Advances in Pain Research and Therapy.* 557–82. Eds. J. J. Bonica *et al.* Raven Press, N.Y.


APPENDIX II

1. Yaryura-Tobias, J. A., B. Heller, H. Spatz, and E. Fischer. 1974. Phenylalanine for endogenous depression. *J. Ortho. Psychiat.* 3(2): 80–81.

2. Fischer, E., B. Heller, and A. N. Miro. 1968. B-Phenylethylamine in human urine. *Arzneim. Forsch.* 18: 1486.

3. Fischer, E., H. Spatz, J. M. Saavedra, H. Reggiani, A. N. Miro, and B. Heller. 1972. Urinary elimination of phenylethylamine. *Biol. Psychiatry* 5(2): 139–47.

4. Mosnaim, A. D., E. E. Inwang, and H. C. Sabelli. 1974. The influence of psychotropic drugs on the levels of endogenous 2-phenylethylamine in rabbit brain. *Biol. Psychiat.* 8(2): 227–34. Whalley, C., A. D. Mosnaim, and H. C. Sabelli. 1973. 2-Phenylethylamine in rabbit brain and liver: Its synthesis, metabolism and role in the action of imipramine, pargyline and marihuana. *Pharmacologist* 15(2): 258.

5. Fischer, E., B. Heller, M. Nachon, and N. Spatz. 1975. Therapy of depression by phenylalanine. *Arznein. Forsch.* 25(1): 132.

6. Spatz, H., B. Heller, M. Nachon, and E. Fischer. 1975. Effects of D-phenylalanine on clinical picture and phenylethylaminuria in depression. *Biol. Psychiat.* 10(2): 235–39.

7. Beckman, H., M. A. Strauss, and E. Ludolph. 1977. DL-phenylalanine in depressed patients: an open study. *J. Neurol. Trans.* 41: 123–34.

8. Fisher, E., H. Spatz, J. M. Saavedra, H. Reggiani, A. N. Miro, and B. Heller. 1972. *op cit.*

9. Beckman, H., D. Athen, M. Oleanu, and R. Zimmer. 1979. DL-phenylalanine versus imipramine: a double-blind controlled study. *Arch. Psychiat.Nervenkr.* 227: 49–58.

10. Heller, B. 1978. Pharmacological and clinical effects of D-phenylalanine in depression and Parkinson's disease. In: *Modern Pharmacology-Toxicology, Noncatecholic Phenylethylamines,* Part 1. Eds. A. D. Mosnaim and M. E. Wolf. New York, Marcel Dekker, pp. 397–417.

11. Spatz, H. and N. Spatz. 1978. Urinary and brain phenylethylamine levels under normal and pathological conditions. In: *Modern Pharmacology-Toxicology, Noncatecholic Phenylethylamines,* Part 1 edited by A. D. Mosnaim and M. E. Wolf. New York, Marcel Dekker. pp. 447–74.

12. Heller. 1978. *op cit.*

13. Borison, R. L., P. J. Maple, H. S. Havdala, and B. I. Diamond. 1978. Metabolism of an amino acid with antidepressant properties. *Res. Commun. Chem. Pathol. Pharmacol.* 21: 363–66.

14. Angst, R. C., V. Autenreith, F. Brem, M. Koukkou, H. Meyer, H. H. Stassen, and U. Storck. 1980. Preliminary results of treatment with beta-endorphin in depression. In: *Endorphins in Mental Health Research.* Edited by E. Usclin, W. E. Bunney, Jr., and M. S. Kline. London: Oxford University Press, pp. 518–528.

15. Kline, N. S., C. H. Li, H. E. Lehman, A. Lajtha, E. Laski, and T. Cooper. 1977. Beta-endorphin-induced changes in schizophrenic and depressed patients. *Arch. Gen. Psychiatry* 34: 1111–13.

16. Krebs, E., and J. Roubicek. 1979. EEG and clinical profile of a synthetic analogue of methionine-enkephalin, FK 33-824. *Pharmakopsychiatr. Neuro-Psychopharmacol.* 12: 86.

17. Gerner, R. H., D. A. Gorelick. D. H. Catlin, and C. H. Li. 1982. Behavioral effects of beta-endorphin in depression and schizophrenia. In: *Endorphins and Opiate Antagonists in Psychiatric Research, Clinical Implications.* Edited by N. S. Shah and A. G. Donald. New York, Plenum, pp. 257–70.

APPENDIX III

1. Ehrenpreis, S., R. C. Balagot, J. E. Comaty, and S. B. Myles. 1978. Naloxone-reversible analgesia in mice produced by D-phenylalanine and hydrocinnamic acid, inhibitors of carboxypeptidase A. In: *Advances In Pain Research and Therapy,* Vol. 3, edited by J. J. Bonica, *et al.,* pp. 479–88. Raven Press, New York.

2. Ehrenpreis, S. 1982. D-phenylalanine and other enkephalinase inhibitors as pharmacological agents: implications for some important therapeutic application. *Subst. and Alc. Actions/Misuse* 3: 231–39.

3. Ehrenpreis, E., J. Greenberg, and J. Comaty. 1977. Mechanism of post-tetanic blockade of transmission in guinea pig longitudinal muscle: Evidence for involvement of prostaglandin and enkephalin. *Pharmacologist* 19: 190–94.

4. Ferreira, S. H. and M. Nakamura. 1979. II Prostaglandin hyperalgesia: the peripheral analgesic activity of morphine, enkephalins and opioid antagonistics. *Prostaglandins* 18(2): 191–200. Ferreira, S. H. and M. Nakamura. 1979. III Prostaglandin hyperalgesia: relevance of the peripheral effect for the analgesic action of opioid antagonists. *Prostaglandins* 18(2): 201–08.

5. Guillemin, R., T. Vargo, and J. Rossier. 1977. Beta-endorphin and adrenocorticotrophin are secreted concomitantly by the pituitary gland. *Science* 197: 1367–69.

6. Millan, M. J. 1981. Stress and Endogenous Opioid Peptides: A Review. *Modern Problems in Pharmacopsychiatry* 17: 49–67.

7. Shanker, G. and R. Sharma. 1979. Beta-endorphin stimulates corticosterone synthesis in isolated rat adrenal cells. *Biochem. Biophys. Res. Comm.* 86(1): 1–5.

8. Oliveras, J. L., J. Bruxelle, A. M. Clorand, and J. M. Besson. 1979. Effects of morphine and naloxone on painful reactions in normal and chronic suffering rats. *Neurosci. Lett.* 53: 263–268.

9. Denko, C. W., J. Aponte, P. Gabriel, and M. Petricevic, 1982. Serum beta-endorphin in rheumatic disorders. *Journal of Rheumatology* 9: 827–833.

# BIBLIOGRAPHY

Akil, H., J. Madden, R. L. Patrick, and J. D. Barchas. 1976. Stress-induced increase in endogenous opiate peptides: Concurrent analgesia and its partial reversal by naloxone. In *Opiates and endogenous opioid peptides,* ed. H. W. Kosterlitz. Amsterdam: Elsevier/North Holland, pp. 63–70.

Alleva, E., C. Castellano, and A. Olivero. 1980. Effects of L-and D-amino acids on analgesia and locomotor activity of mice: their interaction with morphine. *Brain Res.* 198:249–52.

Angst, J., V. Autenreith, F. Brem, M. Koukkou, H. Meyer, H. H. Stassen, and V. Storck. 1980. Preliminary results of treatment with beta-endorphin in depression. In *Endorphins in mental health research,* eds. E. Usdin, W. E. Bunney, and M. S. Kline. London: Oxford University Press, pp. 518–28.

Anselmi, B., E. Baldi, F. Casacci, and S. Salmon. 1980. Endogenous opioids in cerebrospinal fluid and blood in idiopathic headache sufferers. *Headache* 21:294–99.

Antelman, S. M., D. J. Edwards, and M. Lin. 1977. Phenylethylamine: Evidence for a direct, postsynaptic dopamine-receptor stimulating action. *Brain Res.* 127:317–22. Elsevier/North Holland Biomedical Press.

Arrigo-Reina, R., and S. Ferri. 1980. Evidence for an involvement of opioid peptidgergic systems in the reaction to stressful conditions. *Eur. J. Pharmacol.* 64:85–88.

Balagot, R., S. Ehrenpreis, K. Kubota, and J. Greenberg. 1983. Analgesia in mice and humans by D-phenylalanine: Relation to inhibition of enkephalin degradation and enkephalin levels. *Advances in Pain Research and Therapy* 5:289–93. Raven Press, N.Y. Edited by J. J. Bonica *et al.*

Baldessarini, R. J. 1975. Biogenic amino hypothesis in affective disorders. In *The Nature and Treatment of Depression,* eds. F. F. Flack and S. C. Draghi. New York: Wiley, pp. 347–85.

Baldi, E., S. Salmon, B. Anselmi, A. Capellini, G. Capelli, A. Brocchi, and F. Sicuteri, 1982. Intermittent hypoendorphinemia in migraine attack. *Cephalagia* 2:77–81.

Bassett, S. H., R. R. Woods, F. W. Shull, and S. C. Madden. 1944. Parenterally administered amino acids as a source of protein in man. *N. Eng. Med.* 230(4):106–8.

Beckman, H., D. Athen, M. Oheanu, and R. Zimmer. 1979. DL-phenylalanine versus imipramine: A double blind controlled study. *Arch. Psychiat. Nervenkr* 227:49–58.

Beckman, H., M. A. Strauss, and E. Ludolph. 1977. DL-phenylalanine in depressed patients: An open study. *J. Neurol. Trans.* 41:123–34.

Berkowitz, B., A. D. Finck, and S. H. Ngai. 1977. *Neurosci. Abstr.* 3:286.

Bhargava, H. M. 1981. Inhibition of tolerance to human beta-endorphin by a linear and a cyclic peptide. In *Advances in endogenous and exogenous opioids: Proceedings of the international narcotic research conference,* eds. H. Takagi and E. Simon. Tokyo-Kodansha pp. 443–45.

Billig, Harvey E., Jr., and C. Arthur Spaulding, Jr. 1947. Hyperinsulism of menses. *Industrial Medicine* (July): 336–39.

Blankstein, J., F. I. Reyes, J. S. D. Winter, and C. E. Faiman. 1981. Endorphins and the regulation of the human menstrual cycle. *Clin. Endocrinol.* 14:287–94.

Borison, R. L., P. J. Maple, H. S. Havdala, and B. I. Diamond, 1978. Metabolism of an amino acid with antidepressant properties. *Res. Commun. Chem. Pathol. Pharmacol.* 21:363–66.

Bruni, J. F., D. Van Vugt, S. Marshall, and J. Meites. 1977. Effects of naloxone, morphine and methionine-enkephalin on serum prolactin, leutenizing hormone, follicle-stimulating hormone, thyroid-stimulating hormone and growth hormone. *Life Sci.* 21:461.

Buchsbaum, M. S., G. C. Davis, and W. E. Bunney. 1977. Naloxone alters pain perception and somatosensory-evoked potentials in normal subjects. *Nature* 270: 620–22.

Buckett, W. R. 1979. Peripheral stimulation in mice induces short-term analgesia preventable by naloxone. *Eur. Jour. Pharmacol.* 58:169–78.

Budd, K. 1983. Use of D-phenylalanine, an enkephalinase inhibitor, in the treatment of intractable pain. *Advances in Pain Research and Therapy* 5: 305–08. Ed. J. J. Bonica. Raven Press, New York.

Budd, K. 1982, Pain: Theory and management. In *Scientific foundations of anesthesia,* 3d. ed., ed. C. Scurr and S. Feldman. Chicago: Heinemann, pp. 283–90.

Burbach, J. P., E. R. DeKloet, P. Schotman, and D. DeWeid. 1981. Proteolytic conversion of beta-endorphin by brain synaptic membranes. *J. Biol. Chem.* 256(23): 12463–9.

Burrow, G. D. ed. 1977. *Handbook of studies on depression.* New York: Elsevier.

Catlin, D. H., K. K. Hui, H. H. Loh, and C. H. Li. 1977. Pharmacologic activity of beta-endorphin in man. *Commu. in Psychopharmacol.* 1: 493–500.

Cheng, R. S. S., and B. Pomeranz. 1979. Correlation of genetic differences in endorphin systems with analgesic effects of D-amino acids in mice. *Brain Res.* 177: 583–87. Elsevier/North Holland Biomedical Press.

Cheng, R. S., and B. Pomeranz. 1980. A combined treatment with D-amino acids and electroacupuncture produces a greater analgesia than either treatment alone; naloxone reverses these effects. *Pain* 8: 231–36.

Clement-Jones, V., L. McLoughlin, S. Tomlin, G. M. Besser, L. H. Rees, and H. L. Wen. 1980. Increased beta-endorphin but not met-enkephalin levels in human cerebrospinal fluid after acupuncture or recurrent pain. *Lancet* 2: 946–49.

Collier, H. O. J., and A. C. Ray. 1974. Morphine-like drugs inhibit the stimulation by E prostaglandins of cyclic AMP formation by rat brain homogenates. *Nature* 248: 24–25.

Conlay, L. A., T. J. Maher, and R. J. Wurtman. 1981. Tyrosine increases blood pressure in hypotensive rats. *Science* 212: 559–60.

Coupar, I. M. 1978. Inhibition by morphine of prostaglandin stimulated fluid secretion in rat jejunum. *Br. J. Pharmacol.* 63: 57–60.

Denko, C. W., J. Aponte, P. Gabriel, and M. Petricevic. 1982. Serum beta-endorphin in rheumatic disorders. *Journal of Rheumatology* 9: 827–833.

Dewey, W. L. 1982. Structure-activity relationships. In *Endorphins: chemistry, physiology, pharmacology and clinical relevance,* eds. J. B. Malick and R. M. Bell. New York: Marcel Dekker, pp. 23–56.

Donzelle, G., L. Bernard, R. Deumier, M. Lacome, M. Barre, M. Lanier, and M. B. Mourtade. 1981. Curing trial of complicated oncologic pain by D-phenylalanine. *Anesth. Analg.* (Paris) 38: 655–58.

Duggan, A. W., S. M. Johnson, and C. R. Morton. 1981. The distribution of receptors for enkephalin and morphine in the dorsal horn of the cat. In *Advances in endogenous and exogenous opioids; Proceedings of the international narcotic research conference,* eds. H. Takagi and E. J. Simon, Tokyo: Kodansha, pp. 208–10.

Duggan, A. W., J. G. Hall, and P. M. Headley. 1977. *Br. J. Pharmacol.* 61: 399–408.

Dupont, A. et al. 1982. Relationship of opiate peptides to neuroendocrine functions. In *Endorphins and opiate antagonists in psychiatric research,* eds. N. S. Shah and A. G. Donald. New York: Plenum Medical, pp. 99–126.

Ehrenpreis, S. 1982. D-phenylalanine and other enkephalinase inhibitors as pharmacological agents: Implications for some important therapeutic application. *Subst. and Alc. Actions/Misuse* 3:231–39.

Ehrenpreis, S., R. C. Balagot, J. E. Comaty, and S. B. Myles. 1979. Naloxone-reversible analgesia in mice produced by D-phenylalanine and hydro-cinnamic acid, inhibitors of carboxypeptidase A. In *Advances in Pain and Research Therapy* 3: 479–88. Raven Press, N.Y. Ed. J. J. Bonica *et al.*

Ehrenpreis, S., R. C. Balagot, S. Myles, C. Advocate, and J. E. Comaty. 1978. Further studies on the analgesic activity of D-phenylalanine (DPA) in mice and humans. In *Endogenous and exogenous opiate agonists and antagonists,* ed. E. Leony Way, Elmsford, N.Y.: Pergamon, pp. 379–82.

Ehrenpreis, S., J. Greenberg, and J. Comaty. 1977. Mechanism of post-tetanic blockade of transmission in guinea pig longitudinal muscle: Evidence for involvement of prostaglandin and enkephalin. *Pharmacologist* 19: 190–94.

Ehrenpreis, S., J. Greenberg, and K. Kubota, and S. Myles. 1981. Analgesic properties of D-phenylalanine, bacitracin and puromycin in mice: Relationship to inhibition of enkephalinase and beta-endorphinase. In *Advances in endogenous and exogenous opioids: Proceedings of the international narcotic research conference.* Eds. H. Takagi, and E. J. Simon. Tokyo: Kodansha-Elsevier, pp. 279–81.

Elkins-Kaufman, E., and H. Neurath. 1948. Kinetics and inhibition of carboxypeptidase activity. *J. Biol. Chem.* 175: 893–911.

Elkins-Kaufman, E., and H. Neurath. 1949. Structural requirements for specific inhibitors of carboxypeptidase. *J. Biol. Chem.* 178: 645–651.

Emrich, H. M., P. Vogt, and A. Herz. 1982. Possible antidepressive effects of opioids: Action of buprenorphine. *Ann. N.Y. Sci.* 398: 108–12.

Ferreira, S. H., and M. Nakamura. 1979. II-Prostaglandin hyperalgesia: The peripheral analgesic activity of morphine, enkephalins and opioid antagonists. *Prostaglandins* 18: 191–200.

Ferreira, S. H., and M. Nakamura. 1979. III-Prostaglandin hyperalgesia: Relevance of the peripheral effect for the analgesic action of opioid antagonists. *Prostaglandins* 18(2): 201–8.

Fischer, E., B. Heller, and A. N. Miro. 1968. Beta-phenylethylamine in human urine. *Arzneim-Forsch* 18: 1486.

Fischer, E., B. Heller, M. Nachon, and N. Spatz. 1975. Therapy of depression by phenylalanine. *Arzneim-Forsch*. 25: (1)132.

Fischer, E., H. Spatz, J. M. Saavedra, H. Reggiani, A. N. Miro, and B. Heller. 1972. Urinary elimination of phenylethylamine. *Biol. Psychiatry* 5(2): 139–47.

Fox, A. 1983. Aloe vera's $B_{12}$—A new discovery. *Total Health,* 5(4): 48–51.

Fox, A. 1982. The Beverly Hills **Medical** Diet. Bantam Books, N.Y.

Fox, A. 1983. Resistance to Disease Through Nutrition—Part II Phenylalanine. *Let's Live*. Nov. 1983, pp. 16–23.

Fox, A. 1984. Aloe Vera, An Ancient Favorite. *Slimmer.* Aug. 1984, p. 14.

Garzon, J., R. Moratalla, and J. Del Rio. 1980. Potentiation of the analgesia induced in rats by morphine or [D-Ala²]-met-enkephalinamide after intubation of brain type B monoamine oxidase: The role of phenylethylamine. *Neuropharmacology* 19: 723–29.

Genazzani, A. R., F. Facchinetti, M. G. Ricci-Danero, D. Parrini, F. Petraglia, R. LaRosa, and N. D'Antona. 1981. Beta-lipotropin and beta-endorphin in physiological and surgical menopause. *J. Endocrinol. Invest.* 4: 375–78.

Genazzani, A. R., G. Nappi, F. Facchinetti, G. Micieli, F. Petraglia, G. Bono, C. Monittda, and F. Savoldi. 1984. Progressive impairment of CSF beta-endorphin levels in migraine sufferers. *Pain* 18: 127–33.

Gerner, R. H., D. H. Catlin, D. A. Gorelick, K. K. Hui, and C. H. Li. 1980. Beta-endorphin. Intravenous infusion causes behavioral change in psychiatric inpatients. *Arch. Gen. Psychiatry* 37: 642–47. N. S. Shaw and A. G. Donald. Plenum, N.Y.

Gerner, R. H., D. A. Gorelick, D. H. Catlin, and C. H. Li. 1982. Behavioral effects of beta-endorphin in depression and schizophrenia. In *Endorphins and opiate antagonists in psychiatric research, clinical implications,* New York: Plenum, pp. 257–70.

Giardina, W. J. 1974. Analgesic properties of phenylethylamine and phenylethanolamine in mice. *Pharmacology* 12: 1–6.

Goldstein, A., S. Tachibana, L. I. Lowrey, M. Hunkapiller, and L. Hood. 1979. Dynorphin-(1-13), an extraordinarily potent opiod peptide. *Proceedings of the national academy of sciences,* Washington, D.C. 76: 6666.

Guillemin, R., T. Vargo, and J. Rossier. 1977. Beta-endorphin and adreno-corticotrophin are secreted concomitantly by the pituitary gland. *Science* 197: 1367–69.

Halbreich, U., and J. Endicott. 1981. Possible involvement of endorphin withdrawal or imbalance in specific premenstrual syndromes and postpartum depression. *Medical Hypothesis,* 7: 1045–58.

Hambrook, J. M., B. A. Morgan, M. J. Rance, and C. F. C. Smith. 1976. Mode of deactivation of the enkephalins by rat and human plasma and rat brain homogenates. *Nature* 262: 282–85.

Heller, B. 1978. Pharmacological and clinical effects of D-phenylalanine in depression and Parkinson's disease. In *Modern pharmacology-toxicology, noncatecholic phenylethylamines,* Part 1, eds. A. D. Mosnaim and M. E. Wolf. New York: Marcel Dekker, pp. 397–417.

Hosobuchi, Y. and C. H. Yi. 1978. The analgesic activity of human beta-endorphin in man. *Commun. in Psychopharmacol.* 2: 33–37.

Hughes, J., H. W. Kosterlitz, and F. M. Leslie. 1974. Proceedings: Assessment of the agonist and antagonist activities of narcotic analgesic drugs by means of the mouse vas deferens. *British Journal of Pharmacology* 51: 139–40.

Hughes, J. 1975. Isolation of an endogenous compound from the brain with pharmacological properties similar to morphine. *Brain Res.* 88: 295–308.

Hughes, J., T. W. Smith, H. W. Kosterlitz, L. A. Fothergill, B. A. Morgan, and H. R. Morris. 1975. Identification of two related pentapeptides from the brain with potent opiate agonist activity. *Nature* 258: 577–79.

Hyodo, M., T. Kitade, and E. Hosoka. 1983. Study on the enhanced analgesic effect induced by phenylalanine during acupuncture analgesia in humans. *Advances in Pain Research and Therapy* 5: 577–82. Ed. J. J. Bonica *et al.* Raven Press, N.Y.

Jackson, R. L., S. F. Maier, and D. J. Coon. 1980. Long-term analgesics effects of inescapable shock and learned helplessness. *Science* 206: 91–93.

Jacquet, Y. F., W. A. Klee, and D. G. Smyth. 1978. Beta-endorphin: Modulation of acute tolerance and antagonism by endogenous brain systems. *Brain Research* 156: 396–401.

Jakubovic, A. 1982. Psychoactive agents and enkephalin degradation. In *Endorphins and opiate antagonists in psychiatric research,* eds. N. S. Shah and A. G. Donald. New York: Plenum, pp. 89–97.

Janal, M. N., E. W. Colt, W. C. Clark, and M. Glusman. 1984. Pain sensitivity, mood and plasma endocrine changes in man following long distance running: Effects of naloxone. *Pain* 19: 13–25.

Jervis, G. A. 1938. Metabolic investigations of phenylpyrivic oligphrenia. *J. Biol. Chem.* 126: 305–13.

Kline, N. S., C. H. Li, H. E. Lehmann, A. Lajtha, E. Laske, and T. Cooper. 1977. Beta-endorphin-induced changes in schizophrenic and depressed patients. *Arch. Gen. Psychiatry,* 34: 1111–13.

Knoll, J. 1982. Selective inhibition of type B monoamine oxidase in the brain: A drug strategy to improve the quality of life in senescense. In *Strategy in drug research,* Amsterdam: Elsevier, pp. 107–135.

Kosterlitz, H. W., S. J. Paterson, and L. E. Robson. 1981. Opioid peptides and their receptors. In *Advances in Pharmacology and Therapeutics 2, Volume 1: CNS Pharmacology Neuropeptides.* Edited by H. Yoshida, Y. Hagihara, and S. Ebashi. Pergamon, New York, pp. 3–13.

Krebs, E., and J. Roubicek. 1979. EEG and clinical profile of a synthetic analogue of methionine-enkephalin, FK 33–824. *Pharmakopsychiatr. Neuro-Psychopharmacol.* 12:86.

Laverson, N. H., and E. Stukane. 1983. *Premenstrual syndrome and you.* New York: Simon and Schuster, p. 171.

Levine, J. D., N. C. Gordon, R. T. Jones, and H. L. Fields. 1978. The narcotic antagonist naloxone enchances clinical pain. *Nature* 272: 826–27.

Levine, J. D., N. C. Gordon, and H. L. Fields. 1978. The mechanism of placebo analgesia. *The Lancet* 281: 654–57.

Levine, S. Z., M. Dann, and E. Marples. 1943. A defect in the metabolism of tyrosine and phenylalanine in premature infants. III. Demonstration of the irreversible conversion of phenylalanine to tyrosine in the human organism. *J. Clin. Invest.* 22: 551–60.

Lewis, R. J., and R. L. Tatken, eds. 1980. Registry of toxic effects of chemical substances, Vol. 1, DHHS (NIOSH) Publication No. 81-116, p. 98, no. A47533000. Washington, D.C.

Li, C. H., D. Yamshiro, L. F. Tseng, and H. H. Loh. 1977. Synthesis and analgesic activity of human beta-endorphin. *J. Med. Chem.* 20: 325–28.

Liebowitz, M. R., et al. 1983. Biochemical effects of deprenyl. *Psychopharmacology Bulletin* 19(3): 336–39.

Lipman, J. J., B. E. Miller, K. S. Mays, W. C. North, S. Karkera, and W. L. Byrne. 1981. CSF endorphin levels in chronic pain patients and in patients before and after a placebo pain relief. In *Advances in endogenous and exogenous opioids: Proceedings of the international narcotic research conference,* eds. H. Takagi and E. J. Simon. Tokyo: Kodansha-Elsevier, pp. 315–317.

Lipton, M. A., A. DiMascio, and K. F. Killam. 1978. *Psychopharmacology: A generation of progress.* New York: Raven Press.

Loh, H. H., L. F. Tseng, E. Wei, and C. H. Li. 1976. Beta-endorphin is a potent analgesic agent. *Proc. Natl. Acad. Sci.* 73: 2895–96.

Madden, S. C., and G. H. Whipple. 1946. Amino acids in the production of plasma protein and nitrogen balance. *Am. J. Med. Sci.* 211: 149–56.

Madden, S. C., S. H. Basset, J. H. Remington, F. J. C. Martin, R. R. Woods, and F. W. Shull. 1946. Amino acids in therapy of disease. Parenteral and oral administrations compared. Surg. Gynecol. and Ob. 82: 131–43.

Mayer, D. J., D. D. Price, and A. Rafii. 1977. Antagonism of acupuncture analgesia in man by the narcotic antagonist naloxone. *Brain Research* 121: 368–72.

Millan, M. J. 1981. Stress and endogenous opioid peptides: A review. *Modern Problems in Pharmacopsychiatry* 17: 49–67.

Mosnaim, A. D., E. E. Inwang, and H. C. Sabelli. 1974. The influence of psychotropic drugs on the levels of endogenous 2-phenylethylamine in rabbit brain. *Biol. Psychiat.* 8(2):227-234.

Mosnaim, A. D., and M. E. Wolf, eds. 1978. Noncathecholic phenylethylamines. *Modern Pharmacology and Toxicology, Vol. 12.* New York: Marcel Dekker.

Nakano, S., and E. Ikezono, 1981. Effects of electroacupuncture on the levels of endorphins and substance P in human lumbar CSF. *Advances in endogenous and exogenous opioids,* eds. H. Takagi and E. J. Simon. Tokyo, Kodansha-Elsevier; pp. 312–14.

Oliveras, J. L., J. Bruxelle, A. M. Clorand, J. M. Bessan. 1979. Effects of morphine and naloxone on painful reactions in normal and chronic suffering rats. *Neurosci. Lett.* 53: 263–68.

Oyama, T., T. Jin, R. Yamaya, A. Matsuki, N. Ling, and R. Guillemin. 1981. Intrathecal use of beta-endorphin as a powerful and analgesic agent in man. In *Advances in pharmacology and therapeutics II: Vol. 1, CNS pharmacology of neuropeptides,* eds. H. Yoshida, Y. Hagihara, and S. Ebashi. Elmsford, N.Y.: Pergamon, pp. 39–43.

Panerai, A. E., A. Martini, D. Abbate, R. Villani, and G. DeBenedittis. 1983. Beta-endorphin, meta-enkephalin and beta-lipotropin in chronic pain and electroacupuncture. *Advances in Pain Research and Therapy* 5: 543–47. Ed. J. J. Bonica *et al.* Raven Press, N.Y.

Pert, A., R. Simantov, and S. H. Snyder. 1977. A morphine-like factor in mammalian brain, analgesic activity in rats. *Brain Res.* 136: 523–25.

Pert, C. R., and S. H. Snyder. 1973. Opiate receptor: Demonstration in nervous tissue. *Science* 179: 1011–14.

Quigley, M. E., and S. S. C. Yen. 1980. The role of endogenous opiates on LH secretion during menstrual cycle. *J. Clin. Endocrinol. Metab.* 51: 179–81.

Reid, R. H., and S. S. C. Yen. 1981. Premenstrual syndrome. *Am. J. Obstetrics and Gynecol.* 139: 85–104.

Reid, R. L., J. D. Hoff, S. S. C. Yen, and C. H. Li. 1981. Effects of exogenous beta-endorphin on pituitary hormone secretion and its disappearance rate in normal human subjects. *J. Clin. Endocrinol. Metab.* 52: 1179–84.

Risch, S. C., R. M. Cohen, D. S. Janowsky, N. H. Kalin, and D. L. Murphy. 1980. Mood and behavioral effects of physostigmine on humans are accompanied by elevations in plasma beta-endorphin and cortisol. *Science,* 209: 1545–46.

Rose, W. C. 1976. Amino acid requirements of man. *Nutrition Reviews* 34(10): 307–308.

Rose, W. C., B. E. Leach, M. J. Coon and G. F. Lambert. 1955. The amino acid requirements of man. The phenylalanine requirement. *J. Biol. Chem.* 213: 913–22.

Rose, W. C., M. C. Coon, and F. Lambert. 1954. The amino acid requirements of man. VI. The role of caloric intake. *J. Biol. Chem. 210: 331–42.*

*Rose, W. C., D. T. Warner, and W. J. Haines. 1951. The amino acid requirements of man. The role of leucine and phenylalanine. J. Biol. Chem.* 193: 613–20.

Ruther, E., G. Jungkunz and N. Nedopil. 1981. Clinical effects of the synthetic analogue of methionine enkephalin FK 33-824. Paper presented at Third World Congress of Biological Psychiatry, Stockholm (abstract).

Sabelli, H. C., R. L. Borison, B. I. Diamond, H. S. Havdala and N. Narasimhachari. 1978. Phenylethylamine and brain function. *Biochemical Pharmacology* 27: 1707–11.

Sabelli, H. C., J. Fawcett, F. Gusovsky, J. Javaid, J. Edwards and H. Jeffries. 1983. Urinary phenyl acetate: A diagnostic test for depression? *Science* 220: 1187–88.

Sabelli, H., and A. D. Mosnaim. 1974. Phenylethylamine hypothesis of affective behavior. *Am. J. Psychiatry* 131: 695–99.

Sandler, M., C. R. J. Ruthven, B. L. Goodwin, and A. Coppen. 1979. Decreased cerebrospinal fluid concentration of free phenylacetic acid in depressive illness. *Clin. Chem. Acta.* 93: 169–71.

Sandler, M., C. R. J. Ruthven, B. L. Goodwin, G. P. Reynolds, V. A. R. Rao, and A. Coppen. 1979. Deficient production of tryamine and octopamine in cases of depression. *Nature* 278: 357–58.

Shanker, G., and R. Sharma. 1979. Beta-endorphin stimulates corticosterone synthesis in isolated rat adrenal cells. *Biochem. Biophys. Res. Comm.* 86(1): 1–5.

Spatz, H., B. Heller, M. Nachon, and E. Fischer. 1975. Effects of D-phenylalanine on clinical picture and phenylethylaminuria in depression. *Biol. Psychiatry* 10(2): 235–39.

Spatz, H., and N. Spatz. 1978. Urinary and brain phenylethylamine levels under normal and pathological conditions. In *Modern pharmacology, toxicology, noncathecholic phenylethlamines, Part 1*, eds. A. D. Mosnaim and M. E. Wolf. New York: Marcel Dekker, pp. 447–74.

Sved, A. F., J. D. Fernstrom, and R. J. Wurtman. 1979. Tyrosine administration reduces blood pressure and enhances brain norepinephrine release in spontaneously hyperactive rats. *Proceedings of the National Academy of Sciences, Washington, D.C.* 76(7): 3511–14.

Takeshige, C., M. Murai, M. Tanaka, and M. Hachisu. 1983. Parallel individual variations in effectiveness of acupuncture, morphine analgesia and dorsal PAG-SPA and their abolion by D-phenylalanine. In *Advances in Pain Research and Therapy.* 5 pp. 563–69. Ed. J. J. Bonica *et al.* Raven Press, N.Y.

Terenius, L., and A. Whalstrom. 1975. Morphine-like ligand for opiate receptors in human CSF. *Life Sci.* 16: 1759–64.

Thomas, P. K. 1974. The anatomical substration of pain. Evidence derived from morphometric studies on peripheral nerve. *Can. J. Neurol. Sci* 1: 92–97.

von Knorring, L., F. Johansson, B. G. Almay. 1982. The importance of the endorphin systems in chronic pain patients. In *Endorphins and opiate antagonists in psychiatric research: Clinical implications,* eds. N. S. Shah and A. G. Donald. New York: Plenum, pp. 407–26.

Wang, H. L., and H. A. Waisman. 1967. Phenylalanine tolerance tests in patients with leukemia. *J. Lab. Clin. Med.* 57: 73–77.

Wehrenberg, W. B., S. L. Wardlaw, A. G. Frantz, and M. Ferin. 1982. Beta-endorphin in hypophyseal portal blood: Variations throughout the menstrual cycle. *Endocrinology, III:* 879–82.

Whalley, C., A. D. Mosnaim, and H. C. Sabelli. 1973. 2-Phenylethylamine in rabbit brain and liver: Its synthesis, metabolism and role in the action of imipramine, pargyline and marijuana. *Pharmacologist* 15(2): 258.

Wilson, S. P., K. J. Chang, and O. H. Viveros. 1980. Synthesis of enkephalins by adrenal medullary chromaffin cells—Reserpine increases incorporation of radiolabeled amino acids. *Proc. Natl. Acad. Sci.,* 77: 4364–66.

Yaryura-Tobias, J. A., B. Heller, H. Spatz, and E. Fischer. 1974. Phenylalanine for endogenous depression. *J. Ortho. Psychiat.* 3(2): 80–81.

Zeller, E. A., A. D. Mosnaim, R. L. Borison, and S. V. Hoprikar. 1978. In *Advances in biochemical psychopharmacology,* New York: Raven Press.